# ABORTION
## IS A
# BLESSING

# *ABORTION*
# *IS A*
# *BLESSING*

# Anne Nicol Gaylor

PSYCHOLOGICAL DIMENSIONS INC.
NEW YORK, NEW YORK

# Dedication

SEVERAL YEARS AGO in Wisconsin a young high school girl was raped and impregnated by her drunken father. He served a term at Waupun for the crime, but nobody helped the little girl. An honor student, she was forced to drop out of school to become the mother of her father's child.

I do not know whatever happened to that girl, or if her life was salvageable, but I know now that her story is not rare.

To her, and to all the other desperate women our society has treated with such blind and hostile cruelty, this book is dedicated, with gratitude that women finally are becoming free.

# *Acknowledgements*

*I would like to thank*

Patricia Theresa Maginnis for her permission to include four of her incomparable cartoons in this book,

Kay Jacobs Katz for her moving testimony before a Congressional committee, included as an appendix of this book,

Anne Treseder and Beverly Braun for their suggestions and ideas incorporated in NEWS RELEASE— 1984,

my daughter Annie Laurie for her "Foot-in-the Mouth" cartoon and her fashioning of the "Pregnant Proxmire" poster,

my entire family for unfailing patience during five years of an ever-ringing phone,

a new friend, Bea Blair, for her enthusiastic help and encouragement, and an old friend, Hania W. Ris, M.D., for moral support over the years in our work for legal abortion,

my publisher, Robert Wesner, for his concern for women's rights and his willingness to publish a feminist's view of a controversial subject.

—*Anne Nicol Gaylor*
Madison, Wisconsin
April, 1975

# Contents

## Appendices

# Foreword

NEWS RELEASE—1984

Date: *April 1, 1984*

*For Immediate Release*

(Milwaukee) The sobbing parents of a fifteen-year-old rape victim and the physician who performed an abortion for her were sentenced today to life imprisonment by Fetal Rights Judge John Patrick O'Malley under the provisions of the Wisconsin Fetal Rights Act.

The girl herself, raped in January on her way home from an errand for her mother, was sentenced to the Oregon (WI) School for Girls for three years.

"In light of her age, I am showing mercy," Judge O'Malley said. "She could never have arranged an abortion without parental help. However, after her incarceration she will be on probation for thirty years, her presumed span of fertility. Someone who has shown such disdain for life, even though a minor, must be watched closely."

Dr. Jane Beacon, the gynecologist who performed the abortion, is appealing her conviction.

"She'll never win on an appeal," said Prosecuting Attorney Tony Bellano, speaking informally with reporters at the close of the month long trial. "There's no precedent for it. Murder is murder, and this was premeditated murder of the worst kind."

The parents, who have exhausted their financial resources in the current litigation, will start serving their life sentences next week.

Sentences of life imprisonment have become common in Wisconsin for women having abortions, physicians performing them, and those who aid and abet in them since the ratification of the Buckley-Proxmire Human Life Amendment four years ago. That amendment, which bestows full rights of personhood on a conceptus, embryo and fetus, extends homicide and manslaughter laws to cover all abortions except those done to save a woman's life.

To date in Wisconsin no abortions have been done to save a woman's life since the unanimous agreement of a twelve-man panel is required under the Fetal Rights Act.

Judge O'Malley's courtroom is clogged for the remainder of the week with hearings for women charged with minor infractions of the Fetal Rights Act. Most of these involve failure to register pregnancies by the sixth week of gestation. A statewide Pregnancy Monitoring Board was established last year in Wisconsin, but many women are claiming to be unaware of its regulations or unable to meet them. Duties of the Pregnancy Monitoring Board are being carried out principally by the old Selective Service organization. Some communities have Pregnancy Monitoring officers stationed at local post offices. Recently named as Advisory Members to the Wisconsin Pregnancy Monitoring Board are: Cardinal Terrence Cooke, Brent Bozell, Rev. Jesse Jackson, Seals & Crofts, Cesar Chavez, and former President Richard Nixon.

Judge O'Malley's upcoming calendar is crowded with Fetal Rights cases, including alleged attempts at self-abortion, continued use of IUD's (known now to act as abortifacients), inquiries into so-called "spontaneous" abortions which the prosecutors believe were undertaken intentionally, and the charges against a Milwaukee clergywoman, Rev. Ellen Norreo, who is accused of referring a Milwaukee woman for an abortion to Japan where the procedure remains legal.

Next week a trial will start before Judge O'Malley, involving a twenty-eight-old mother of six, who is being charged with failure to register her pregnancy, with the alleged intention of aborting herself by a prolonged motorcycle ride, undertaken to do herself sufficient bodily harm to cause abortion.

"This woman put her selfish concerns above the rights of the new person within her," exclaimed Prosecuting Attorney Joseph O'Hanrahan. "This is a nation under God. She and all women like her must be punished. All human life is sacred. 'Vengeance is mine,' saith the Lord."

Encouraged by the success of the Buckley-Proxmire Human Life Amendment, a national movement is now under way to extend the legal rights of personhood to the egg and the sperm.

"The precedent is already there," said Mrs. Michael Francis Ryan, president of the Wisconsin Voice of the Unconceived. "The wording in the Buckley-Proxmire Amendment says the person is protected at 'every stage of its biological development,' and surely this includes the egg. We should have no trouble ratifying an amendment to protect the innocent egg and the innocent sperm in Wisconsin, since Wisconsin law always has regarded contraception as 'indecent.'

"Think of the babies lost because of contraception and sterilization," Mrs. Ryan continued, "Think of the innocent, immature life of the egg and the sperm. Someone must speak out for this unrepresented segment of society that cannot speak for itself.

"Of course ours is not a Catholic movement," she added, "but an ecumenical movement. Every child has the right to be conceived."

---

So it can't happen here?

This book was written because it *can* happen here! The right of a woman to choose legal abortion can be taken away—unless the political efforts of religious extremists seeking to ban abortion through constitutional amendment are countered in Washington D.C. and in state capitals.

The historic, compassionate Supreme Court ruling of Jan. 22, 1973, freed millions of women from sexual servitude and from the dangerous, traumatic search for illegal abortions. This ruling, our country's greatest step forward in social and moral progress since the abolition of slavery, must be protected politically by the activism of individuals who write letters to legislators, attend hearings, visit their Congresspersons, and support groups working to keep abortion safe and legal.

For the past five years I have been in daily contact with women seeking abortions, and I have learned, as I could in no other way, of the tragedies that have been avoided because abortions are available. The stories of the hundreds of women that I have counseled personally, and the thousands of women from all over the country that I have talked to on the phone, have resulted in my clear understanding that abortion is a positive thing, a cure, a blessing.

I have become impatient not only with those religious zealots who tiresomely hiss "Murderers," but with those apologists who, while granting the right to abortion, insist that somehow a woman must feel guilt and remorse. I have come to suspect that the persons who refer to abortion as "a tragic option," or "a terrible alternative," hold allegiance not to women's freedom but to a male-dominated world gone by.

While recognizing that safe, sure contraception is a preferred alternative to abortion, I deal daily with the casualties of our "modern" contraceptive methods, and I recognize reality, that abortion does what contraception does not necessarily do: it works. I am further aware of the rigid, religious prohibitions against contraception of which certain women remain the victims. I know that far too many women in our country find contraception unavailable, especially if they are young or poor. I know that the teen-aged victim of incest can hardly be expected to be practicing contraception. And I have never heard of a rapist who used condoms.

In a sense I have been privileged to see firsthand the great need for abortion, and I have written this book to share my feelings and experiences so that others might come to see why abortion is a blessing, not only for women but for society. It is my hope that those who read this book will join in the effort to keep abortion safe and legal until that idealistic time when education, medical research, and human behavior combine to make abortion obsolete.

# "How Did You Get Involved?"

IN MY VOLUNTEER WORK for abortion in the past few years, I have been asked repeatedly, "How did you happen to become involved?" I usually have answered the question superficially because to answer it adequately would require a lengthy dissertation. But, in reality, it began in grade school with Ethel, who was impregnated, reportedly, by her brother.

Like most of the little girls I knew I regarded babies very highly, and as a farm child with few nearby playmates I used to daydream about someone leaving a baby on our doorstep for me to play with, as happened with delightful frequency in the books I read. The idea that a baby, or a pregnancy, could be unwanted did not occur to me until an older student in our one-room country school became pregnant.

Ethel was a shy, large, rather slow girl from a tenant farmer's huge family. It was not too long after the first shocked whispers about her pregnancy began to circulate that she dropped out of school, never to return. For poor young Ethel, age fourteen, biology was destiny.

There were a few forced marriages in our high school and the usual dropouts for unwed, unwanted pregnancies.

And no wonder! Sex education for female students consisted of "a woman from the state" who came to the high school every other year or so to talk to the junior and senior girls for a class hour. We learned somehow—no explicit words were ever used—that intercourse could result in pregnancy, but we were not told how to prevent pregnancy. The sessions were acutely embarrassing, both for the red-faced woman from the state and for her audience. Questions very quickly turned to the safer subjects of menstruation, dating, and "going steady." The lesson we really learned was that sex was something you didn't discuss.

In my years as a student at the University of Wisconsin in Madison, one young woman's sad story impressed me forever with the futility of enforced pregnancy. At nineteen, pretty and popular (crucial traits in the 1940's), she was raped by an older man, an acquaintance of her family, and pregnancy resulted. Her parents sent her to the Twin Cities to complete the pregnancy, but her newborn baby was placed for adoption privately, with a Madison couple.

Tragically, after a few months it was learned that the baby was mentally retarded. The adoptive parents did not want the child, it could not be placed elsewhere, so it was institutionalized for a lifetime of care at public expense. And all of it was so unnecessary. The young woman's life was shadowed needlessly with physical and mental suffering; the product of rape was an abnormal child *nobody ever wanted.*

On my first visit to an obstetrician's office after my marriage, I sat across the waiting room from a mother and daughter. The sadness on their faces was obvious to anyone, as was the young girl's pregnancy. She seemed at most eleven or twelve years old, and she was the first *pregnant child* I had ever seen. I thought then, as I do now, that it was grossly inhumane that a child should have to become a mother. Babies having babies is a cruelty beyond compare. We do not let our immature animals breed, but our girl children—well, "that's fate."

2

Several years ago, when my husband and I lived in the University area of Madison, I was awakened one night by a rising and falling sound. At first I thought it was a mechanical sound, some eerie kind of siren. Then, sleepily I decided that it might be an animal, that perhaps a dog had been hit by a car and was crying in pain. Finally, fully awake, I realized with horror that I was listening to a woman screaming. I watched from the front windows of our home as an ambulance came to a nearby house to take her away. Her pain was so great that the eerie, animal screams were audible even after the ambulance doors had closed behind her. I learned the next day that the young woman, unmarried and pregnant, had attempted to abort herself.

During the 1960's so many tragic stories came to my attention, both in the press and from friends. There were occasional little items in the papers about a newborn baby found floating in the Rock River, and babies left dead or alive in shopping bags, in theatres, and wooded lots. A social worker told me of her attempts—unsuccessful—to secure an abortion for a mother of eight retarded children, to prevent the birth of a ninth retarded child. There was an illegitimacy explosion in the sixties with a consequent dismaying backlog of babies waiting for adoption— even the white-skinned, blue-eyed, golden-haired babies waited in those days.

One incident in the late sixties crystallized my thoughts on abortion, and resulted in my conviction that it must become legal. A teen-ager in Wisconsin, pregnant without her family's knowledge, delivered her baby at home alone at night. Distraught with pain and fear, she panicked when the baby began to cry and killed it, stabbing it with a pair of scissors.

Nine months can be an eternity when you are young. I could only shudder at the thought of a young girl carrying that secret burden for that length of time, and then going through the agony of first childbirth without anyone to help her. By her tragic action she had told us in the most

3

pathetically eloquent way she could that this was an unwanted child. I knew that regardless of how abortion was looked upon, it was infinitely humane compared to the horror of unwanted pregnancies.

In 1967 as editor of a suburban weekly newspaper, I wrote the first editorial ever written in Wisconsin, calling for abortion law reform. I repeated this call for reform in a letter published in a national medical newspaper. In response, a New York physician wrote urging me to become active and join the Association for the Study of Abortion (ASA), one of the country's early abortion reform groups founded by professional people in New York. It was the first of a half-dozen groups concerned with freedom to choose abortion that I was to join. Soon, Edith Rein, a Milwaukeean who pioneered abortion reform and referral in Wisconsin, contacted me, encouraging me to start a chapter in Madison of her organization, the Wisconsin Committee to Legalize Abortion.

And so I became involved.

# The Phone Calls Begin

A MILWAUKEE PHYSICIAN, Sidney Babbitz, was arrested in the fall of 1969, and charged with performing a criminal abortion in his offices. His lawyers took his case to federal court, challenging the constitutionality of Wisconsin's abortion law, which was similar to most of the abortion laws across the country, in that abortion was legal only to save a woman's life. Penalties went as high as fifteen years in prison.

On a blustery January day in 1970, this case was heard in the federal courtroom in Milwaukee before a three-judge federal panel composed of former Wisconsin governor John Reynolds, former Illinois governor Otto Kerner, and Myron Gordon.

As I sat in that courtroom listening to the arguments, I could not help reflecting that here was a case of the *utmost importance* to women, yet no women were heard. The judges, of course, were men. The opposing attorneys were men, as were the witnesses. Only in the courtroom audience were there any women and, by law, they were mute.

The panel's verdict was handed down in March of 1970. Unanimously the judges agreed Wisconsin's abortion law was unconstitutional.

With their ruling and the consequent publicity about it, my phone started to ring, with women calling wanting to know where to go for abortions. Five years and several thousands of calls later, the phone still rings, but how the times have changed!

Everyone who called cried in the beginning. And well they might.

One doctor, Alfred Kennan, a gynecologist at the University of Wisconsin Hospital in Madison, accepted some patients, but the hospital had a meager quota, high prices ($600 for an early abortion), and the stipulation of two letters from other physicians that the abortion was necessary to preserve the woman's life. Despite these hurdles, that route took care of a few of the women who called me, and I referred some others to Milwaukee hospitals which had essentially the same red tape and high costs. Abortion, court ruling or no, was available only if someone had lots of determination and cash money, and started to search early enough in her pregnancy so that she could wait the month or more she might have to, for a hospital appointment.

In the spring of 1970 I referred about forty of the women who could not be helped in Wisconsin to Mexico. Through Bob McCoy, a Minnesota pioneer in abortion reform, I learned of a clinic in Mexico City that charged $300 and that Bob had checked out for safety and considerate treatment of women. Abortion was illegal in Mexico (still is), but the practitioners reportedly paid off the chief of police and were able to operate unmolested.

The women I referred to Mexico flew from Chicago at a round-trip cost of $226. They had to spend two nights in Mexico City and while there stayed at the San Jorge Hotel, which was built for the Olympics. They were advised to take about $40 spending money to cover the hotel, their meals, and sightseeing.

Dr. Ponce, who owned the Mexico City clinic, did abortions by the dilation and curettage method, under general anesthesia.* Women were at the clinic for a morning or

*(See Appendix A for a discussion of abortion methods.)

6

afternoon. The extra twenty-four hours in Mexico City was both a health precaution and helped women avoid airport questioning by the immigration people. It did occur to me that patrons having to stay an extra day in Mexico also benefited the hotel, although their rates were relatively modest. Since abortion was illegal, women flying in and out of Mexico in a short time could be subject to questioning about the reason for their trip. We told everyone, if asked, merely to say they were on a short vacation.

Those of us referring women were still under the spell of the old ideas about abortion—that it was a major medical effort with some of the risks of brain surgery—so I was delighted and astonished when one of my early referrals, an intrepid woman, phoned in her report to me. She said she had the abortion in the morning, flew back to Chicago in the afternoon—ignoring the two day stay—and took a bus home to Eau Claire, Wisconsin, at night, about an eight-hour trip. She felt fine, she said, "just a little tired." Most women reported some discomfort following abortion —nausea from the anesthetic or cramping, similar to menstrual cramping.

Bob McCoy had prepared a sheet of general information about the hotel, meals, and sightseeing, with a little map of the hotel area, information on converting money, cab and subway guidance, and recommendations of restaurants. Places to get carryouts and inexpensive food were suggested, as well as the "Focolare," one of the city's finest restaurants with dinners costing about $8.00. Women were cautioned to watch out for automobile traffic, a far greater hazard than abortion, and aggressive males, a universal hazard.

Someone from the clinic called for the women at the San Jorge Hotel, and chauffeured them for their appointments. In the directions, with medical and clinic information, Bob McCoy and Dr. Ponce had written " . . . after you have been interviewed, you will go upstairs and put on a surgical gown. You may wish to take slippers with you to keep your feet warm." When I first read this in the directions, I almost cried. I was fresh from pleading with Wis-

7

consin doctors to accept especially desperate patients for abortion and had found almost all of them totally indifferent to the plight of any woman, yet here were men who were concerned not only that women should have abortions, but also that they should not have cold feet!

Most of the women I referred to Dr. Ponce phoned in their reports, and without exception they liked him. Ponce was a first name, I believe, not a family name, but it was the only name we knew him by. He interviewed each woman before the abortion and checked out each patient before she left. Somehow, despite the assembly line, he managed to make each woman feel his concern for her.

The clinic was sanitary and comfortable. Here is an excerpt from one report sent in from an out-of-state referral.

> Things were really good down in Mexico City. Everything happens so fast there is almost an aura of fantasy. The clinic (more like a mansion really) is very nice and comfortable.
>
> There were about seventeen women there the morning I had the D & C done, plus some in the afternoon. They get you up right after and feed you fruit and drink and cookies right away— helps take your mind off the cramping.
>
> Some of us went sightseeing that afternoon. Mexico City is really nice, and I had no trouble at all with any facet of the journey or my stay there.

One young woman, with whom I spent quite a bit of time before she flew down because she was unusually tense and unhappy, came back calm and relaxed. She gave me all the factual information including the friends she made and the sights she saw, and then added, somewhat apologetically, "You know, in a way it was almost fun." I don't know when a remark has left me more cheerful. I thought of all the women who had been forced to go into dark alleys and back rooms and deal with perverted, unskilled, unsanitary practitioners, and I could only rejoice that for

8

some women abortions were being done in a safe setting with supportive people, and that the whole trip could be "almost fun." Civilization has been a long time finding women.

My referrals in the spring and summer of 1970 had been pretty much happenstance; the women happened to learn that I knew where safe abortions were being done. I had appeared on several radio and television talk shows on the abortion issue, and women called after hearing these or after seeing my name in news stories, or reading letters I wrote to editors.

One letter to me prompted the decision to establish a formal, advertised service. It read:

July 27, 1970

Dear Mrs. Gaylor:

Since I received your letter July 9th many things have happened, and I now have the chance to sit down and thank you for everything you did.

I had written you requesting information on abortion in the State of Wisconsin after reading your letter to the editor in the *Appleton Post Crescent.*

The next day my fiancé came up and he got on the phone immediately. The first doctor he contacted from your list was able to help us. We were in Milwaukee the next morning. I had a physical, and arrangements were made for my admittance to the hospital in less than two weeks. The treatment I received, both the hospital care and personal, was more than I could have hoped for. Things haven't been left at that, since I'm under the doctor's care for a future checkup.

I am still amazed at how easily and swiftly things went and how well everyone treated us. If only it weren't so hard to find out about these things in the first place. Of the women I talked to in the hospital, the majority seemed to have found out about the availability of an abortion quite by accident and only after much agonizing about what they were going to do.

In the future if there is anything I can do to help your organization, I will be more than happy to do so. After what has been done for me and my fiancé, it would be small payment for getting our lives back to normal again and being able to enjoy being engaged and making future plans that won't be marred by the reality of having to bear an unwanted child and making many more lives than our own miserable.

Thank you again.

E.S.

This letter and its reference to women finding out quite by chance and after much worry convinced me to become more visible. I had joined the Zero Population Growth (ZPG) organization because of its supportive position on abortion, and I asked the board of directors of the Madison chapter if they would consider funding advertising of a service, if I would use my own phone number and handle the calls. They readily agreed.

The first ad, placed in the classified "Personal Interest" section of Madison's two daily papers on August 12, 1970, read: "ABORTION is legal and available in Wisconsin. If your doctor won't help, contact the Zero Population Growth Referral Service." The ad included the ZPG post office box and our home phone number. The response was immediate. By the end of the month, in less than three-weeks time, we had received ninety-three calls and the phone has not stopped since.

Ours was the first advertised service in Wisconsin, possibly in the Midwest, and calls came in from surrounding states as well. When *Playboy* magazine listed several referral numbers around the country, including ours, in one of its issues, I was deluged with calls for months from as far away as Maine, Virginia, Arkansas and points west. *Playboy* readers called at all hours—one, two and three-thirty A.M. I announced to my patient family that, contrary to popular opinion, *Playboy* readers rarely went to bed—they phoned people all night long.

There are not too many occasions for chuckling when you are handling abortion referrals, but our children supplied a couple. After a few calls from the first ad, one of our sons remarked, "Well, we don't have to answer 'hello' anymore. We can just say, 'How far along are you?' " And, after the United States Supreme Court decision in 1973, legalizing abortion, when my phone calls jumped to 140 in a single week, the kids came out one day with an unusual observation. Commenting on my practice of answering the phone by number, 238-3338, and my chances for survival, they said, "We've decided on your epitaph. We're going to put on your tombstone, 'Here lies 238-3338.' "

Since I couldn't be home all of the time, other Madison ZPG women helped with the service. In all, a couple of dozen women have handled calls, for periods of anywhere from a few weeks to a few months time, using their home phone numbers as back-up numbers in our ads. Especially helpful in the early days were Gail Winkler, then president of ZPG in Madison, Donna Anderson, Martha Maxwell and Barbara Banchero.

I kept a log of telephone calls for the referral service, primarily to keep a record of the number of calls, where they were coming from, ages of the women, and notes on contraceptive failures. Since so many days the calls came thick and fast, the entries really were very sketchy, and some days I resorted to a simple tally. Typical entries read: "Rockford, 20, kids 3-2-6 months, pregnant on foam." "Chicago, 29, kids 8-6-4-2-1, went off the pill, could pay $100 down." "Holmen, Wis., 25, sounded 50, three children, problems with hemorrhaging, needs abortion and wants tubal ligation, 'can't get any help around here,' gave Milwaukee hospitals." "Richland Center mom for 15-year-old, needs D & C, gave UW Hospital."

Any ideas I may have harbored about a typical abortion

11

patient vanished when the phone began to ring in earnest. The stereotype of the abortion candidate is that of a young, single woman, working or in college. I heard from that stereotype, but I heard almost as often from the married woman. Almost daily women called who could not take care of the children they already had, or who had grave medical problems compounded by repeated pregnancies. From the beginning I heard regularly from victims of rape and victims of incest. I heard from teen-agers who were pathetically young, who were children themselves by every standard except that of fertility.

Very early in my referral experience a doctor with whom I was pleading for help told me, "Well, you can refer me the really desperate cases." I said to him what had become only too terribly clear to me, "They are all desperate."

Letters came in to the ZPG post office box, too, and the first one, so typical of those to follow, was from rural Wisconsin and written on a scrap of yellow paper.

> Dear Sirs: Please send me information on the laws that would cover our situation. My wife and I have nine children from 16 to 2 in age. We own our own home, but I have to work 70 hours a week to keep things going. Is there any doctors that will at least talk to us on abortion? Any information will be helpful because my wife is three months along again.     H.B.

Abortion became legal in New York state on July 1, 1970. Miraculously, the pro-abortion groups there had forced a reform law through their legislature, and the dramatic victory meant that New York would go from a situation where they had one of the most restrictive abortion laws in the world, to a situation where they had one of the most liberal.

The immediate effect was a logjam. Women from all over the country went to New York for abortions. Clinics and hospitals were booked out of sight, and it was the end of 1970 before waits were down to a somewhat reasonable two-week delay. Quality and costs varied greatly at the different facilities, and women pretty much took potluck the first few months. Later, through Clergy Consultation Service on Problem Pregnancies, a non-profit New York City clinic was established with a charge of $150, soon to be reduced to $125. I also referred to the Eastern Women's Center when it opened in 1971, charging $150.

Here are a couple of typical reports from that period.

Dear Anne:

It's fantastic being able to control your own self and destiny. Yesterday I flew from O'Hare to LaGuardia in New York and had an abortion at the office you suggested. The aspirator is relatively painless and one of the doctor's assistants, a very understanding girl, stands by you for the entire procedure, which, in my case, took less than fifteen minutes.

The fee for me was $100 and certainly the most worthwhile $100 I have ever spent. Thank you so much for your most valuable referral.

K.T.

Dear Mrs. Gaylor:

I previously contacted you for referrals concerning abortion clinics. I was admitted to the Women's Medical Group in New York in January.

I was admitted to a room where my blood test and urine specimen were obtained. My friends were directed to a waiting room downstairs. I sat in the waiting room approximately two hours talking with girls having appointments also. Then a counsellor came and took me to an office where I was given pills and relaxed. We talked about the abortion procedure, post-operative feelings, complications, my feelings and fears, for about an hour.

Then she took me upstairs again where I had

13

the operation in fifteen minutes, rested a half hour and went home.

The counseling was excellent and she stayed with me through everything, even assisting the physician. She, too, had had an abortion, which made for greater understanding.

If complications should arise, their collect phone number is given to each woman, along with brochures containing abortion post-op and complication information and birth-control methods. It was worth far more to me than $150.

L.S.

Madison got its own abortion facility, the Midwest Medical Center, in February, 1971, the only outpatient clinic in the country between the east and west coasts. It was opened by Dr. Alfred Kennan, its only doctor, and it was almost immediately swamped with patients. Dr. Kennan did abortions by vacuum aspiration, utilizing gentle suction to empty the uterus and employing a local anesthetic, in contrast to the traditional hospital procedure of dilation and curettage done under general anesthesia. Although the clinic could accept only a tiny fraction of the women seeking appointments, it was a haven for about ninety to one hundred patients per week in the early months, a schedule later increased to 120–125 weekly.

The clinic had been open for about eleven weeks when Madison police in a sudden, Gestapo-like raid, closed it. The raid seemed particularly insane, in light of the federal court ruling that Wisconsin's old abortion statute was unconstitutional, and the permanent injunction that had been issued, saying no Wisconsin doctor could be prosecuted for doing an early abortion.

About this time Gail Winkler of ZPG and I were subpoenaed to appear for an interrogation conducted by the attorney general's office, on behalf of the State Board of Medical Examiners, who were after Dr. Kennan's license. Their methods and their questions had us wondering if we lived in Wisconsin or a banana republic.

Both Gail and I received our subpoenas during the dinner hour at night, telling us to appear before the Board early the next morning. Although the hearing had been scheduled for some time, and we were obviously busy people, the Board saw fit to give us only a few hours notice. There was little time to contact an attorney—Gail never had had occasion to consult one before, and the lawyer who had handled some business affairs for me happened to be out of town. There was not even time to go to the law library to read the law we were being subpoenaed under. Fortunately, a friend phoned to suggest an attorney, whom we met for the first time outside the Board of Medical Examiners' offices early the next morning. And we stayed outside. Two uniformed *armed* guards stood at the door, and we were told we would be called when we were needed. We waited in the hot sun for almost three hours. The attorney, young and kind, whose name I don't remember and who never sent us a bill, had come with a law book under his arm, and in checking our subpoenas discovered we had been subpoenaed under a portion of the law requiring that a judge be present to grant us immunity. When finally—hot, tired and sunburned—we were admitted to the presence of the Board, our lawyer asked the prosecutor from the attorney general's office, who was presiding, where the judge was. The attorney general's assistant seemed taken aback, inplying that this was an informal, friendly little session and no judge was needed. When our attorney pointed to the citation on our subpoena and the corresponding number in the statute book, the attorney general's assistant said that the subpoena was in error, that a different part of the law was really being referred to, that it was a "typographical error." Our lawyer responded that since the subpoena said what it did, he could only advise us to answer questions before a judge, and since no judge was present, he was advising us not to answer questions at all.

Gail and I were interrogated separately, and both of us took the Fifth Amendment to a long series of inane questions. At the end we were told we would be "bound over to

15

court to answer before a judge," an event that never took place. The interrogator apparently was trying to link the ZPG Referral Service to Dr. Kennan's clinic, so that Dr. Kennan might be accused of advertising. There was no link. Not only did the Referral Service precede the clinic by half a year, but no able doctor who did abortions in 1971 had any need to advertise. All he had to do was open, and the whole country beat a path to his door.

After six weeks of court maneuvers, when Attorney General Robert Warren had been put down at every court level, the clinic finally reopened, but the cost to the 324 women who had appointments when it was closed has never been tabulated. I spoke personally with about forty-five of these women and I am still haunted by their stories, their anguish, and their helplessness. My loathing for the men who perpetrated these harassments does not lessen with time, although I am happy to report that District Attorney Gerald Nichol was defeated for reelection in 1972. Attorney General Robert Warren, however, was appointed to the post of federal judge in Wisconsin's Eastern District, Richard Nixon's last official act before being forced from the Presidency. *It figures!*

The chapter that follows is an account of the raid written originally for the ZPG-Madison newsletter, and later expanded into an article for the *ZPG National Reporter*. The chapter titled "The Victims," which also appeared in the *National Reporter*, was my testimony before the Judiciary Committee of the Wisconsin Assembly, which held hearings on abortion the day after the clinic reopened.

3

# The Raid*

IN THE FACE OF . . . HOSTILITY, and almost in the shadow of the Capitol, one courageous doctor chose to open an outpatient abortion facility. Dr. Alfred L. Kennan, a gynecologist, resigned his academic post as professor at the University of Wisconsin Medical School in January, 1971, and on February 1 opened Wisconsin's first outpatient clinic, the Midwest Medical Center in Madison.

The legal basis for his action was a decision of a three-judge federal court, sitting in Milwaukee, which had said in March, 1970, that the state of Wisconsin could not deprive a woman of making her private decision on whether or not to carry an unquickened fetus. The court followed its decision some months later with a permanent injunction, saying that the state of Wisconsin might not prosecute "any Wisconsin doctor" for performing abortions in early pregnancy. This injunction, upheld by the Circuit Court of Appeals in Chicago, seemed a plausible legal basis for proceeding.

Soon after its opening in February, the clinic was

*This chapter first appeared as part of an article in the July, 1971, *ZPG National Reporter*. Originally titled "Abortion in Wisconsin?", it is reprinted with permission.

17

booked three weeks ahead, about as far ahead as abortion appointments realistically can be made. About a hundred patients a week were accepted, also a maximum for a one-doctor clinic. Although there were rumblings of official and unofficial displeasure, including a march on the Dane County District Attorney's office by a group of so-called "right-to-lifers," demanding that the clinic be closed, it operated unmolested for two and one-half months.

Then, quite suddenly, on Monday, April 19, at three o'clock in the afternoon, several policemen and women descended on the clinic. Bursting into offices and procedure rooms, they grabbed all records and equipment, and forcibly took with them a terrified seventeen-year-old girl, ignoring a clinic counselor's plea that she be allowed to accompany her. Asked if they were arresting the girl, they said they were, and she was taken to a Madison hospital where she was forcibly examined against her will. Minors in Wisconsin have no rights.

Although the raid was conducted on Monday, formal charges were not made until late Wednesday, when Dr. Kennan, two nurses, and the Center's two counselors were charged with criminal abortion.

The clinic's phones were wild on Tuesday with all five lines tied up by patients trying to check appointments and asking what they should do. Eight or nine women came in to the clinic with their friends or family on Tuesday, unaware of the raid. One of the first patients had been driving since three o'clock in the morning to be on time for her appointment. An afternoon patient had driven from the Mankato area in Minnesota, some 300 miles away. None of the patients could be notified by the clinic in advance, because the appointment book had been taken in the raid. Over 300 women had made appointments.

The raid was ordered by Dane County District Attorney Gerald Nichol, on the basis of a complaint by a Minnesota woman. The woman had phoned Madison police the week before to say she believed her runaway daughter was on her way to Madison for an abortion. Madison policemen picked up the girl and her friend after they left the clinic on the Friday before the raid, taking them to the station for questioning. A search-and-seizure warrant was then secured in county court and the raid was on.

Liberal Madison was stunned and angered. Even many who had not spoken previously for abortion condemned the ruthless tactics utilized in the raid. An editor of Madison's liberal newspaper, the *Capital Times,* pointed out that the clinic was not a hidey-hole operation, but an open, aboveboard, highly visible clinic, providing safe abortions done by an eminently qualified specialist in pleasant supportive surroundings.

A rally outside the district attorney's office at noon on the day following the raid drew 200 people, many of them ZPG'ers. On Thursday, the day of the arraignment of the clinic's personnel, about 350 supporters of the clinic were on hand, at ZPG's behest, to continue the peaceful protest.

Groups of doctors, medical students, nursing students, and clergymen joined to sign and release formal publicized protests. ZPG petitions circulated and rapidly were filled.

New York clinics stretched crowded calendars to take dozens of the clinic's cancelled patients, with rates adjusted in many cases.

And then, the Monday after the raid, the action moved to Federal Judge James Doyle's court where Dr. Kennan had applied on April 20 for injunctive relief. Judge Doyle heard arguments for an order to restrain the state from prosecution of the clinic staff, and to convene a three-judge federal panel to hear the case. A pregnant woman, who had an appointment at the clinic, joined in with a legal class action on behalf of all women who had planned to use the clinic.

Spectators overflowed all chairs and benches and were allowed to take seats in the jury box. The audience was orderly except at two points—once when District Attorney Gerald Nichol entered the courtroom (what did he expect?), and again when an assistant attorney general,

Mary Bowman (can she be for real?) said: "If giving birth to unwanted children is irreparable harm, then women in Wisconsin and all over the country have been surviving it for over 120 years."

There was an air of buoyancy in the courtroom at the close of the proceedings. Judge Doyle's kind manner and his words "You will have my decision by noon tomorrow" sent clinic-boosters home to sleep well for the first time since the raid.

He didn't quite make his noon deadline, but it didn't matter because Judge Doyle's decision was to restrain the state from its prosecution, order the equipment returned to the clinic, and call for the three-judge panel to rule on the law.

Friends of the clinic didn't get a chance to celebrate however, because other legal actions followed before the clinic could open, including an effort by the State Board of Medical Examiners (in effect, an arm of the attorney general) to suspend Dr. Kennan's license, a civil action instigated by the attorney general and filed in county court, and a try by the city to keep the clinic closed on a zoning charge. These legal obstacles took a few weeks to beat down, with able assists from Judge Doyle in the form of restraining orders. The clinic finally reopened on May 24, 1971.

Its future is very uncertain, but its past is clearly quite noble, and ZPG-Wisconsin gave its Humanitarian Award, 1971, to Dr. Alfred L. Kennan for "his courage and compassion in founding the Midwest Medical Center."

4

# *The Victims*\*

WHAT HAPPENS when an abortion clinic closes? When Dane County District Attorney Gerald Nichol ruthlessly closed Madison's Midwest Medical Center on April 19, 1971, he set into motion a chain of tragic events whose total effect may never be known. Lawmakers, so prone to investigate everything, could be investigating these tragedies, but of course they are not. At least they can listen; they can listen to what happened to one Wisconsin girl.

This girl had an appointment at the Midwest Medical Center the week it was closed. She and her boyfriend had read about the clinic in their local papers, and although they had only a little money they were able to arrange an appointment for a partial fee. When the clinic was raided, they were all but paralyzed, because they had no knowledge of where else to turn. At first they procrastinated, then the boy made several calls to hospitals and doctors, but they were all abrupt with him. Those who talked to him at all talked about the high cost of a hospital abortion, the need for parental consent, the legal uncertainties. They suggested no other alternatives of places to go and the young couple's despair deepened.

\*Testimony given at the abortion hearing of the Judiciary Committee, Wisconsin Assembly, May 25, 1971

The boy and girl had come to each other from backgrounds of parental rejection; the girl had run away from her home. They had both been hurt, they had been unhappy in their home life. In each other they seemed to find some measure of security and acceptance, of uncritical love, something they had never had.

Although the boy had no thought of abandoning the girl, she became terribly depressed. She could only think that each day she was getting farther and farther along into this unwanted pregnancy, and what a terrible burden she was becoming to the boy. He was the only one she had to cling to and she was afraid. So one night, without the boy's knowledge, she took a last desperate way out of her problem. She took a wire coat hanger and jabbed it into her uterus. Toward morning, when the pain became too much to bear, she told the boy what she had done and he went to get help for her.

Now because he was very young and frightened, he did not call the logical people to call in an emergency—a doctor or a hospital. You will remember they had rejected him before. He did not call the police because he actually feared he and his girl would be arrested. He phoned collect to a clergyman in a town a hundred miles away, who was the only person he felt he could trust, and this man put him in touch with a counselor in his own city.

The counselor came out and convinced the boy that his fears of legal retribution were overblown, and that the girl was in very serious condition. She helped him take her to a hospital.

But they were too late. The girl had punctured her uterus with the hanger, she had bled excessively, and she died in the hospital a few hours later.

Last night I talked to the counselor who was with the girl when she died, and she asked me to convey a message to you. Tell the legislators, she said, that it is a terrible thing to watch a young girl die, and to know that her death was unnecessary, a total waste. Tell them how terrible it is that anyone should have to lose her life because of fear, because everyone who could help her was too intimidated by our unjust law to give her the help she needed. Let them know about this girl's family, who last saw her warm and alive and now will see her always as something dead, to be carried out and disposed of. Tell them about this boy who had to be physically restrained from destroying himself when he realized his girl was dying. Don't let them sit there and debate abortion, without knowing the tragedies that occur when abortion is not available. Let them know about this girl—one girl's death is one too many. . . .

When the Midwest Medical Center was closed in April, 324 women had appointments there. Where did they all go? What could they do?

Many of them who could afford to go to New York City went to clinics and hospitals there. A handful were accepted in Wisconsin hospitals.

Five or six of them, without much money, wound up in an old house in Milwaukee where, they reported, a drunken pervert made sexual advances toward them before giving them botched abortions. At least two of these women were hospitalized in serious condition.

And what of the others? Consider one case, a Madison woman of twenty-three. The woman is not married, she never has been married. She already has three children, five, three, and one. She is enrolled in a program to help her to complete her schooling and learn a trade, so that she may become employable. This woman could barely afford Madison's clinic, even at an adjusted rate of $58. She could never afford to go to New York City. Now past the time when abortion is simple, safe, and relatively inexpensive, she will be quitting her training. She will have a fourth unwanted child that will have to be supported to maturity by others. And her last hope to be anything but a breeding machine may be gone forever.

And what about the Rock County woman, the married mother of eight children, who cries throughout conversations because she is so desperate about another unwanted pregnancy? She could afford the $50 the clinic had arranged to charge her—there is no one else in the country she could go to with her $50.

And what about the young Milwaukee woman, married, with three children, five, four, and three? Her husband is unemployed. She works—for $1.26 an hour in a burger joint. She is pregnant—she cannot afford to be pregnant—her family needs her income. She is too late now for an outpatient abortion—what is she to do? What is her family to do? What is our society going to do when it cannot take care of the unwanted children already born?

Wisconsin women are going to have abortions. If they have enough money they are going to travel to states where it is available. If they do not, they are going to seek out the incompetent, unsafe abortionists, or attempt to abort themselves.

This legislature cannot stop the tide of abortion reform or the acceptance by women of abortion. You can only succeed in making it dangerous or inconvenient or expensive for them. In the cases where you are able to make it impossible to get, you will be adding the burden, both social and financial, of unwanted children to our state.

Women are going to be free. They are going to determine their reproductive lives as they wish; this is the essence of dignity and personal freedom. No one can know better than a woman herself whether it is best for her to bear a child. In a world that cannot possibly take care of the children it already has, what folly to force unwilling women to bear unwanted children.

Abortion is going to be legalized in Wisconsin. It is not a question of *if,* it is a question of *when.* Humane men and women will work to legalize it now, so that women's suffering and death may be avoided.

# 5

# *Why Abortion?*
# *More Letters*

OVER THE YEARS a few hundred letters have been written to the ZPG Referral Service in Madison, requesting abortion referral information.

Most of them are brief: "I would like information on abortions. I am forty-eight, married, and for health reasons cannot bear another child." Or, "Please send me some (*any*) information on abortion. I cannot phone you as it's a party line." And, "Read your personal interest ad in the paper that abortion is legal and available. Would you please send us more information on this. I'm married and we have seven children now." And, "We would very much appreciate any information you might be able to provide concerning abortion for the mother of a family that is presently sufficient."

Parents also wrote:

> Can you please help us? We have an eighteen-year-old daughter that is seven weeks pregnant. .
> . She is four months from graduating from high school and if the school finds out she is pregnant they will kick her out. She is also accepted at a college and wants to go very bad.

Now that abortion is legal in Wisconsin we thought we could get a doctor to do it. Everyone we talked to refused. . . . We have to have some help soon and make some definite plans for her, or she might look for help by herself, and I'm afraid of what would happen. She is our only child, and we don't want anything to happen to her. Please try and help us. . . .                J.B.

Desperation is conveyed in a great many of the letters.

Since I've never done this before I really don't know what to ask. I am pregnant, five weeks, and I definitely cannot have a baby. My family and my job would be over. . . . Please, I am almost going crazy. I don't know what to do any more. I need some kind of information very soon.                D.G.

I am twenty-four and found out yesterday I am pregnant. . . . I have made up my mind an abortion is the only answer as the man I am pregnant by is the guy I have been going with for four years, but in that four years he has only worked three months and I know he won't change. Also, he is half black, and even if I wanted a baby, it wouldn't be fair to the baby. It is hard enough making it in this world without being part black and without a father and without a decent home.

Anyway, I have made up my mind that it's the only solution and want it done as soon as possible. Please help me as I haven't told anyone except you. Please call me collect as soon as you get this letter. . . . I need help soon!                L.C.

Please, please help me. I am absolutely sure I am pregnant, but I cannot possibly have a baby. It would not only postpone indefinitely completion of my much loved college work, but my having a child would bring untold problems to my parents, both of whom are prominent members of this community. . . . The man is at his home, 300 miles away, so I am as usual when it comes to an abortion, alone. Please help me.                L.J.

I found your address in a Planned Parenthood booklet, and I would like to know if you can help somebody like me. I just found out that I am pregnant and I am eighteen and a half and unmarried. I can't tell my parents because it would hurt them too much and also because I am scared. . . . Please help me. I am so scared I don't know what I am going to do.                D.B.

Sometime ago I heard your comments on the radio about legalizing abortion, agreeing with you all the way. I am a widow, fifty years old, and find that I am two months pregnant. I am putting two children through college with one other at home. You could write me or call me, but the only thing in telephoning is that someone would be listening in as they do in a small town. Please try to help me—the sooner the better. Thank you.
                I.G.

Here are a couple of reports.

I had wanted to write you earlier and thank you for your most gracious and kind assistance on the phone. . . . I was truly very desperate and so very sick. . . . The type of surgery was absolutely unexpected since I was given total anesthesia, thus feeling no pain or cramps. I had expected from my past experience six years ago in Chicago to be in great pain. . . . Again, my deep thanks for your efforts on women's behalf.                S.G.

I want to thank you for your prompt reply to my letter and for the information given me. I don't think I have ever felt so down in my life, but when I arrived at the clinic in Madison they made me feel so at ease and they were so very kind to me that I shall never forget it. . . .                    N.D.

I think the following letter from a young married woman in rural Dane County is my favorite. Surely no document of its size ever radiated more appreciation, cheerfulness, and good will. The hospital I referred her to required a psychiatric note stating that an abortion was necessary for her life and health, hence the reference to the psychiatrist.

Dear Mrs. Gaylor:

I am writing to inform you that my abortion was a great success.

I went first to the psychiatrist and got a letter the same day I went to him. He was very kind in every respect.

I called the doctor you suggested the same day, and he told me to come to Milwaukee as soon as I could. That doctor is just a fabulous person, and I would recommend him to anyone who has to have an abortion. I went into the hospital the fourth of September, had surgery the fifth and came home the sixth. The surgery was a D & C with a general anesthetic. The hospital was everything a hospital should be: very clean and everyone on the staff was so very nice. I was so impressed by the hospital that I wrote a nice thank-you card to them for the many kindnesses they showed me while in the hospital.

I had no pain after surgery or when I got home. Once in a while I had a slight twinge, but it didn't amount to anything. All I can report about the doctor and hospital is that I can't say enough good things about my experience.

I would like to thank you so very much for
being so nice and willing to help me in my time of
need.                                                    M.R.


This gracefully expressed letter came from a sixteen
year old girl for whom I had scoured the state seeking a
doctor to help her.


Dear Mrs. Gaylor,
    I've wanted to write so many times before, but
never knowing what or how to say thank you,
which seems hardly enough to one who has done
so much, I have put it off until now. For this, I am
very sorry.
    I have so much to be thankful for and all of this
I owe to you. This summer would have been so
difficult for me if you hadn't taken the time to
help me. Instead these past few months have
been so wonderful. I find myself appreciating
even the little things that I am able to do, knowing that without your help I couldn't be doing
much except hiding at home.
    Next month I am going to visit my father. I
know I wouldn't have been able to face him if I
had been pregnant. You see, he expects so much
of me, as most fathers do of their daughters, and
I just couldn't have hurt him like that. I know I
should have thought of that a long time ago, but
unfortunately I didn't stop to think about anyone
but myself.
    Some people say that sooner or later I'll regret
having had an abortion, but I know that if I had
gone through with my pregnancy there would
have been much, much more to regret.
    Now I can start over, a much wiser and I hope,
more mature person. So many girls don't get a
second chance. Thank you for mine.          B.H.

And, last, a most untypical note from a harried young man seeking information for his girlfriend:

Dear ZPG: I am the dummy who meant to send you a request for information and sent you my sociology lecture notes instead. Here is the letter I meant to send.                                                        J.B.

# 6

# *The Unforgettables*

ONE OF THE COUNSELORS at the Midwest Medical Center in Madison phoned me late one Friday afternoon to say a woman with two babies had come into the clinic at closing time. She had come up on the bus from St. Louis and needed a place to stay, since she had neither the energy nor money to return to St. Louis and come back to Madison the next week.

Our daughter, Annie Laurie, started putting her room to rights to receive company, and I drove over to the clinic to pick up the patient, Nancy Belle, and her babies.

Nancy was black, from the St. Louis ghetto, and she told me she had missed the bus she intended to catch, hardly surprising when you're traveling with two babies and have no one to help you. She couldn't decide whether to return to her apartment or wait for another bus, but she thought she might never get up her courage again, so she waited for the next bus with her babies, a boy two, and a girl, eight months.

On our way home I learned she had two other children who were staying with relatives in another city, one four years old and one three.

Nancy was twenty-one. Although she was bright and

31

quick and wanted to work, the only job she had ever held was as a temporary clerk in a warehouse. She had dropped out of school during her second year of high school when she became pregnant, and at that point, if not earlier, her life's script was written for her.

Nancy was only repeating what she knew. She was one of eight or nine children from a home that had never had a permanent father. Hers was the life style of the young, single woman as she knew it. Only Nancy was a little more courageous than most. She had heard that there was an abortion clinic in Madison, so when she found out she was pregnant again, she took her babies, got on a bus, and came to get an abortion.

Nancy lived in an especially dreary and dangerous section of St. Louis. She said she never went out without a gun in her purse and tried never to go out at night at all. Despite the gun, she had been robbed once of her rent money. Like most of her friends, she subsisted on Aid for Dependent Children (ADC).

We borrowed a crib from neighbors for her baby girl to sleep in, and she told us it was the first time any of her four babies had ever slept in a crib. She thought our old-fashioned kitchen was the height of style, and she had never tasted some of the ordinary foods we had. Her health showed the effects of five years of chronic childbearing. Thin and frail, she suffered from an ulcer and an asthmatic condition, both triggered by pregnancy. Part of her weekend with us she nursed a throbbing tooth.

We liked Nancy very much and we loved her babies, but we worried about her two-year-old boy. She never smiled at him the whole weekend, and whenever she spoke to him, it was to admonish him. He seemed to be the focal point on which she could release all her tensions and frustrations, and when he wet himself, quite natural for a two-year-old in strange surroundings, she spanked him with a viciousness quite out of proportion.

So here was Nancy Belle with children aged four, three, two, and eight months. No one had ever said to her, when you have babies so close together you not only harm yourself, you cheat them in health and you cheat them in brains and you cheat them in love. And what could she have done if she had known?

Had there not been an abortion clinic in Madison and had Nancy Belle not had the extra gumption to get there, she would have had five children at age twenty-one, or perhaps the ghetto abortionist might have had another victim.

We sent a couple of letters and cards to Nancy—she had no phone—but we didn't hear from her for about a year. She had never been able to stay on the pill because of the bad side effects, so she used her Medical Card to have an intrauterine device (IUD) inserted a few weeks after her abortion. Then the IUD caused a serious uterine infection and she had to be hospitalized for a week.

Now she was writing because she was pregnant again, only, happily, in the year's interval abortion had been legalized by the United States Supreme Court and she could be referred to a safe clinic near her home.

Her dilemma, in a sense the dilemma of women everywhere, has me perpetually outraged with our society, which has money to supply much of the world with armaments, to fly to the moon, to print millions of unwanted pamphlets on strange subjects, to engage in all manner of inane bureaucratic wheelspinning, yet will not give priority to the search for contraception that is safe and reliable.

An important postscript: Dr. Kennan of the Midwest Medical Center in Madison did Nancy's abortion for free as he has done so many others. Although the clinic was closed on Saturdays at that time, he came in that Saturday morning to do the abortion for her.

When I drove Nancy to catch her bus back to St. Louis after her weekend with us, I glanced over at her little boy sitting on my daughter's lap. Still under the effect of a spanking for his bad toilet habits, he was subdued and tearful. When I lifted him on to the bus, he turned and clung to my hands, a tiny victim in the pathetic cycle of

33

unwanted children producing more unwanted children.

*   *   *

Eileen was never more to me than a small voice on the other end of the long-distance line, but as her story unfolded she seemed to symbolize the great wrongs that doctors, hospitals, church and state have inflicted on women.

She was in her late thirties, in a *fifteenth* pregnancy. She had eight or nine living children; her other pregnancies had resulted in stillbirths or miscarriages. She had all the ailments associated with excess childbearing—varicose veins, pernicious vomiting, kidney and bladder problems. Although her last four births had been by Caesarean section, she had been denied the tubal ligation she asked for at the time of her last delivery.

For readers unfamiliar with these terms a Caesarean section is a major operation, in which a large incision is made through a woman's abdomen and uterus to deliver a baby when she cannot deliver normally. At the time a Caesarean is done, since the abdomen is already open, it is very simple for a doctor to do a tubal ligation or sterilization, cutting the Fallopian tubes, so the woman's eggs no longer reach her uterus. Because of the large wound, a Caesarean patient is usually hospitalized ten days. After leaving the hospital she must return to her doctor regularly for checkups, until the wound is totally healed. Most physicians recommend tubal ligations after three Caesareans, since there is risk in future pregnancies of rupture of the much-scarred uterus. Such a rupture usually results in death. A tubal ligation done at the time of a Caesarean section does not add to the woman's hospital stay, to the surgical risk, or to her bill; so it is practical from every standpoint to have it done at the time of a Caesarean section.

Eileen and her husband both worked to support their large family. A latecomer to the pill because of her Catholicism, she had had to give it up because it made her constantly nauseous. Now she was pregnant again. She couldn't afford to be pregnant because she needed to work. She could not face another pregnancy physically, let alone another Caesarean. Her Catholic upbringing left her poorly prepared to deal with abortion, but she was calling because she knew, as I knew, that she was fighting for her life.

The Midwest Medical Center was booked three weeks ahead at that time, but Dr. Kennan agreed to take her as an extra patient. He came back at night to do the abortion for her, working her in very promptly since she was already at ten weeks, the cutoff for the suction abortion method.

So much of my time in the past few years has been spent helping people pick up the pieces of their lives that never should have been pieces in the first place. Any woman, let alone a woman who has had four Caesareans, has every right to have a tubal ligation if she wants one, and the doctor and hospital who deny it to her should have their respective licenses revoked. Eileen did not want an abortion any more than Nancy wanted an abortion; no woman *wants* an abortion. But women will continue to have abortions until society recognizes their need for sure, safe contraception, and until all hospitals offer access to permanent birth control through sterilization.

Among my referrals has been one other woman in a fifteenth pregnancy. She, like Eileen, had had several of the pregnancies end in stillbirth or miscarriage; she, luckily, had had only *two* Caesareans. It is a terrible commentary on the calibre of the medical profession in Wisconsin that these women should have had to endure what they endured. They both had obstetrical histories that would have elicited sympathy from a stone, yet their physicians would not help them. These abominable doctors would rather have their women patients suffer and risk death than do a simple, safe, sensible tubal ligation for them.

\* \* \*

I have referred so many women with so many great problems—medical, financial, social—that it is difficult to sort out the unforgettables. In a sense, as individuals, they are all unforgettable. I have referred twelve- and thirteen-

35

year-olds for abortions and I have referred grandmothers, the oldest fifty-two. Women I've referred have represented every social and economic class and they have ranged in attitude from the organized, composed matron who could say, "Cost is no problem," to the totally disorganized teen-aged girl who sobbed, "I'm pregnant and I don't want a baby and I don't have any money and my boyfriend has left town and what am I going to do?"

It saddened me that so many of the women seeking abortions had physical problems which meant that they never should have been pregnant at all. So many women had diabetes, or heart conditions, or epilepsy. One woman had two children both with serious heart defects, and could expect another child to have the same disability. Another woman who called from St. Louis had a blind baby, and her doctor had told her the chances were fifty-fifty that this pregnancy would result in another blind child. Bone-marrow disease was a defect in another family that the woman could expect to transmit to a child. For all of these women it was an undeniable blessing that there were oases of help in Madison, Wisconsin and New York City, where they could go for safe, legal abortions.

The callers I couldn't help are unforgettable too; many of these were mothers of large families. There is a woman in Madison who phoned me when she was twenty-four and had five children. After the birth of the fifth child she got birth-control pills from a doctor, but her husband found them and threw them away, saying no one was going to tell him how many children he could have. When she phoned, she was four months pregnant. Had we been able to get her into University Hospital in Madison for the late abortion (which we couldn't, since they take only a few and are always booked ahead), there still would have been the problem of husband's consent and money. In New York, where a husband's signature is not so commonly required by hospitals, she would have been accepted, but how could we come up with the large amount of money needed to get her there?

36

Another mother of ten children told me that after the birth of her last baby she wanted to take the pill, but her husband, a staunch Catholic, would not let her. Here was another woman who called too late for outpatient care; we could do nothing for her, since a Madison hospital abortion would have required her husband's signature and financial help. Again, the hassle and expense of going to New York made that out of the question.

One rural woman I referred told me that because of her husband the only birth control method she could use was rhythm, and they had had seven children that way. Her husband was employed only seasonally, so in addition to just not being able to face another pregnancy she was burdened with great financial worries. She had pleaded with her doctor to help her with contraception, but he told her she was "healthy as a horse and could have ten more." She had the abortion, as many mothers of large families have had, without her husband's or her doctor's knowledge.

There was the young woman with four kids, three and one-half, two and one-half, one and one-half and three months. She had begged her doctor to do a tubal ligation at the time of her last delivery, but he had refused her, saying, "Dear, I'm surprised you would even think of it. Anyway, you're only twenty-three." This gem of a physician, the only one in her community, didn't believe in contraception either. Fortunately, she was in time for a clinic abortion.

Some days the phone calls were not only unforgettable, but they made me feel like a Madison outpost for Guinness World Records. One morning I referred a thirty-two-year-old woman with eleven children, all single births. Another woman, twenty-five, had seven children, the oldest six. Besides the six-year-old there were five-year-old twins, a four-year old, three-year-old twins and a ten-month-old baby. One fifteen-year-old girl I referred already had had two Caesareans.

Rape and incest calls were commonplace, but I soon learned that rape by strangers is far less common than rape by relatives. I referred teen-agers impregnated by their fathers, their stepfathers, their brothers, their half-brothers, their brothers-in-law, their uncles and their cousins. There were days when I decided Wisconsin was just one big Peyton Place.

I also made the discovery that a certain amount of rape goes on *within* many marriages. Over the years I talked to a dozen Catholic mothers of large families who said in essentially the same words: "I could do without sex. I would have done without sex rather than take a chance on another pregnancy, but my husband couldn't." Slavery, of sorts, is still with us.

Among my family's unforgettables was the fragile, beautiful African woman who came on the bus from Michigan and stayed with us the night before her early-morning appointment at the clinic. Her husband, a graduate student, would have had to drop out of school if she had had another child.

We remember Francie who came down from northern Wisconsin with her six-months-old baby and stayed at our house. Francie's recollections of her delivery were only too vivid; her doctor did not believe in any anesthetic, and Francie, although she was a strong, athletic young woman, still reacted with terror to the thought of her particularly painful and exhausting delivery, *au naturel.* Since she was obviously in need of reassurance, I told her I knew this doctor with whom she had her appointment, Dr. Dusan Jovanovic, would keep her comfortable during the abortion, but I saw she was still apprehensive. On the way to the doctor's office to pick her up after her appointment, I hoped I hadn't overdone the reassurance; women have such different thresholds of pain. But abortion was easy for Francie. When she saw me she smiled and said, "I didn't feel a thing"—music to my ears.

Once I asked John Carr, who was business manager of the Midwest Medical Center in 1972-73 during its very busiest times, if he had an unforgettable patient. During that time John was seeing about 120 patients a week, all kinds of possibilities. Since I knew that out of every one hundred patients, the clinic could expect two to be victims of rape and three to be victims of incest, I expected him to refer to one of these. Unhesitatingly John said that there was a married couple whom he would never forget. They came in to the clinic from northern Wisconsin and their poverty was very apparent. They had ten children at home. John said they were fat, the unhealthy fat of years of living on surplus starchy foods, and their teeth were rotting from lack of care. His office soon filled with the aroma emanating from stale, unwashed clothes and unwashed bodies. They were nice people, John said. They were well-meaning, likeable people. Yet they were caught in the vicious trap of poverty because they had not been able to stop having babies.

Until now.

# Coping With the Antis: Questions and Answers

THE SHRILLNESS OF THE antiabortion clamor in this country has not lessened with the United States Supreme Court decision in 1973. Those opposed to a woman's right to choose abortion, primarily members of the Catholic Church and various fundamentalist sects, have announced that their ultimate goal is the overthrow of the decision through constitutional amendment. In the meantime, their strategy is to weaken its impact through the passage of unconstitutional bills at the state and national level, which then must go through the long, laborious process of challenge in the courts.

That the antiabortion forces have numbers and money is not in doubt. They have lobbying offices in Washington D.C., and a national monthly newspaper devoted entirely to antiabortion news. They have had the resources to publish antiabortion books and place them in tens of thousands of schools and libraries, to run full page "fetus ads" in newspapers across the country, and to finance public relations gimmickry such as smothering the Capitol in roses signifying "lost lives"—embryonic lives, naturally, not women's lives. Their demonstrations at state capitals and in Washington D.C. have drawn substantial crowds.

The various antiabortion bills and riders, especially those in the restriction of physicians' access to public and private hospitals for purposes of performing abortions and sterilizations, have been somewhat successful.

But their blitz, the big fight, the passage through Congress of an amendment to the Federal constitution to ban abortions, has made only noise, not progress. And hopefully it will continue to spin its wheels, as more individuals and groups speak out on behalf of the right to choose abortion.

Every day that abortion is legal and available in this country new adherents are gained for its continued legality. All Americans, including antiabortionists, have been able to see for themselves that abortion can become a private decision for a woman and her physician, and the world does not fall apart; in fact, it becomes a healthier, kinder, saner, less punitive place. Most counselors, social workers, clergypersons, or members of the medical community who finally deal firsthand with the reality of abortion become quiet converts. That we could return to the useless devastation of women's lives that was the norm before abortion availability seems unthinkable now.

But no freedom ever comes easily, nor is it retained without constant vigilance. Women must work to protect and extend their right to choose abortion. Pendulums swing and the swing toward women's rights could be countered, unless groups supporting women's freedom make it clear once and for all that a woman's uterus is not a political football.

Advocates of the right to choose abortion have too often allowed their opponents' tactics of distortion to go unchallenged. Chronically, antiabortionists represent abortion as involving an elephantine fetus about to walk and talk, when, in truth, the typical abortion has more in common with a menstrual period. With outrageous disregard for truth, antiabortionists have been allowed to portray an embryo or fetus as a person, while the story of the real person involved, the only person involved—the woman

42

who has an abortion—has gone untold. Almost every grass-roots community in America has had the opportunity to see the antiabortionists' distorted, inaccurate, gory slide presentations. Few have had the chance to see a suction abortion performed although these medical movies are available.*

Education, of course, is the answer. The antiabortionists have been allowed to blur the picture but when the focus clears, the legality of abortion will remain secure. Had the proponents of legal abortion had the access to money, to schools and churches, and to the media that the antis have had, the only proponents of a ban on abortions in this country today would be those zealots who oppose not only abortion but contraception, and in the final analysis, sex itself.

Since the controversy goes on, it may be useful to review some talking points in coping with the zealots. In fielding questions on abortion on talk shows and before civic, school and church groups, I have found the antis' questions fall into patterns. Here are some typical questions with answers that worked for me.

QUESTION: *How can your group condone abortion when it is murder?*

Obviously we do not regard abortion as murder. We do not equate an embryo or fetus with a human being. While we recognize that there is everything in a human embryo to produce a person, we know that substantial growth and development are necessary before any person exists. In reality everyone does distinguish between potential and actual existence. You do not insist, for example, that an acorn is an oak tree. If someone drives over an acorn in your yard, you do not rush out and exclaim, "Why did you destroy my oak tree?" Yet there is everything in an acorn to produce an oak tree *except* growth and development. You do not insist that the egg you ate for breakfast was a

*See Appendix D.

43

chicken, yet a fertilized egg has everything in it to produce a chicken *except* growth and development. If you go to the store to buy apples and are given a handful of seeds, you will not pay for apples, even though the storekeeper might argue correctly that indeed apple seeds do produce apples. Just as blueprints are not a completed building, so a human fertilized egg is not a person. A conceptus, an embryo or fetus is potential life. Birth makes babies and a great deal of growth and development must go on before a fetus can sustain life, other than parasitically.

At the end of the second month of development, and most abortions in the United States are performed before the end of the second month, an embryo is approximately an inch in length and weighs one-thirtieth of an ounce. To say that this embryo in its primitive development is a human being is an affront to honesty. Think for a moment what you would do with such an embryo if you had one. You could not rock it, or feed it, or sing to it. All that you could do would be to put it on the shelf because it is an embryo; it is not a baby. It is potential life; it is not a human being.

QUESTION: *I have talked to lots of people who say abortion isn't really legal? Is abortion legal?*

Yes! On January 22, 1973, the United States Supreme Court, by ruling oppressive Texas and Georgia abortion statutes unconstitutional, legalized abortion across the country.

Although abortion may not be *available* in every state, it is *legal* in every state. The only regulation a state may make about abortion in the first three months is to require that it be done by a licensed physician. For the second three months of pregnancy, a state may, if it wishes, say abortions must be performed in hospitals, or similarly regulate conditions protecting the health of the woman. Only in the final three months of pregnancy may abortion be prohibited by state law, and even in that period a woman may have an abortion to protect her life or health.

Don't let any antiabortionist tell you differently!

QUESTION: *How can you support abortion when that unborn child that is murdered might turn out to be another Beethoven or Shakespeare?*

While it is possible that an aborted embryo or fetus might have turned out to be another Beethoven or Shakespeare, it is equally possible it might have turned out to be another Genghis Khan, another Adolf Hitler. As one proponent of abortion has so aptly said, the overwhelming chances are that it would have turned out to be just another Joe Blow. It is possible to speculate endlessly about what might have happened, about the nonexistent.

In our world of almost four billion persons, it is highly probable that a Beethoven or Shakespeare already exists who will never see a piano or learn to read, because the child lives in a Chicago ghetto or Manila slum or Rio de Janiero *favela*. The potential of millions of children already born will never be realized because of malnutrition, illness, and poverty. Antiabortionists, in their obsession with the quantity of life, ignore the quality of life. Their consuming concern for embryos rarely is paralleled by a concern for children already born.

QUESTION: *You say a woman should be able to make this decision for herself. Why shouldn't the father be able to say whether or not an abortion can be done? After all, the child belongs to him, too, doesn't it?*

We believe no woman should have to bear a child she does not want. Compulsory pregnancy compounds problems; it does not solve them. We are against enforced pregnancy no matter who is doing the enforcing—

45

whether it is the state, the church, or an individual man.

From a practical point of view, if a couple does not agree on something as basic and important as having a child, what kind of parents are they going to be? What kind of marriage must they have? At best, they are going to produce a half-wanted child.

And why shouldn't pregnancy be a woman's decision when she contributes so much more to the pregnancy than does the man? An ejaculation, which takes a few seconds, can not be equated fairly with nine months of gestation, and delivery. You must remember that pregnancy is not much fun. For many women, by the time they have quit vomiting they have started to bulge, and the whole process can be nine months of acute discomfort.

If a woman produced one or two eggs in her lifetime then what happened to those eggs would be of great concern, not only to her, but to society. But she doesn't produce one or two eggs, she produces about 400 mature eggs. Obviously they can't all become persons. Clearly society can afford to let her determine for herself which eggs she sees through to personhood.

QUESTION: *I can see abortion in cases of rape or incest or if there is a strong possibility that a fetus is retarded or deformed, but if some sixteen-year-old tart goes out and gets herself pregnant, why should she be able to have an abortion?*

She should have an abortion because no sixteen-year-old girl should have to bear a child. No woman, regardless of age or circumstances, should be forced to have a baby. You are viewing pregnancy and the consequent birth of a baby as punishment. What a wretched reason for a baby to be born! A teen-aged girl who becomes pregnant has a legitimate claim to anyone's sympathy, to any doctor's help. She is physically immature, mentally immature, insolvent, unhappy, her education incomplete. What sense does it make to compel her to become a mother when the safe, simple alternative of abortion is available?

46

QUESTION: *Won't abortion mean fewer and fewer babies to adopt in this country?*

Perhaps, and hallelujah! No woman should have to turn herself into a breeding machine so somebody else can adopt a child. A scarcity of babies to adopt means that so many of the formerly unadoptable—the older children, the black children, the mixed race children, the children with handicaps—are finding homes. Also, there is new pressure to ease the ludicrous restrictions on intercountry adoptions. There are literally millions of homeless children in the world; there are also artificial, bureaucratic barriers keeping them and potential parents apart.

In relation to adoption, it is valuable to contrast our attitudes toward adoptive and natural parents. For years we have insisted that adoptive parents be not too old or too young, that they have stable personalities and even stabler incomes, that they supply references, that they survive group and individual in-depth interviews as to their suitability for parenthood. Yet, on the other hand, we have forced the thirteen-year-old girl, the mother worn out from childbearing, the penniless woman and the woman who is ill—all of whom did not want to be pregnant, none of whom could have got a foot in the door of an adoption agency—to continue pregnancies and to become parents. How ludicrous that we should maintain such lofty standards for parenthood on the one hand, and have absolutely no standards at all on the other.

QUESTION: *Doesn't abortion make women sterile?*

No. Improperly performed abortions may result in cervical damage, sterilization, or even death. But properly performed abortions, especially those done in early pregnancy using a local anesthetic and a suction aspirator, are very safe, several times safer for a woman than childbirth.*

*In 1973 the death rate for women in childbirth in the U.S. was 14/100,000, for abortion 3/100,000. The death rate for first trimester abortion was 2/100,000. Death rates can be expected to decline still further when physicians become more skilled at abortion techniques.

QUESTION: *Don't most people object to the legalizing of abortion? Doesn't the referendum in Michigan prove this?*

Most of the polls done in 1974 show the country about evenly divided on the issue, with those persons favoring legal abortion a few percentage points ahead.

Antiabortionists love to refer to the 1972 Michigan referendum, in which a proposition to legalize abortion was defeated 61–39 per cent, but that particular referendum probably only proves that the Catholic Church has a lot of money. A comparison is useful here. In one of the western states a few years ago a modified ban on cans was proposed and went out to referendum. Polls showed that an overwhelming percentage of the state's voters would favor the referendum and wished to put an end to the waste of basic materials and the unsightliness of scattered cans. Then those who objected to the can-ban got busy. They launched an expensive public-relations campaign deliberately designed to cause apprehension, inferring a can-ban might mean a recession in the state's economy and a consequent loss of jobs. In the end the can-ban, whose backers had spent a small sum, failed.

In Michigan early polls showed 56 per cent of the voters favored legalization of abortion. Opponents, who hired an advertising agency, staged a three-week blitz before the referendum, saturating television throughout the state with antiabortion commercials. As an example of their diligence, they came over to Green Bay, Wisconsin, to place commercials, since Green Bay serves some of the upper peninsula of Michigan. Gory and inaccurate brochures found their way to almost every one's door; one woman reported receiving thirteen pieces by mail and personal delivery. The Catholic Church used its tax-exempt machinery openly for the political purpose of helping defeat a referendum, and of course it won.* Tyranny is always better organized than freedom.

*Detroit Free Press,* March 4, 1973.

48

The lesson to be learned from the Michigan referendum is that advertising campaigns, especially when they are inaccurate, blitz campaigns that are not countered, may sway voters.

It is of questionable constitutionality, of course, to put individual rights out to referendum. It's as undemocratic as letting Alabama and Mississippi decide whether blacks should vote. Basic human rights, including a woman's right to control her own reproductive life, are guaranteed by the Constitution. They are not to be decided by popular referenda or church edicts or male legislatures.

*   *   *

Since I have spoken quite widely in Wisconsin on the abortion issue, people who will be participating themselves in formal discussions or debates on abortion frequently call me, wanting pointers on fielding questions or handling cross fire. Besides touching on the material already discussed in this chapter, I suggest the following:

*Challenge your opponent's vocabulary.* The arguments and materials used by antiabortionists are quite predictable, and to a man or woman, they will use the same vocabulary. All embryos are "children" to them, all women are "mothers," and all men are "fathers." Challenge them! Point out that an embryo or fetus is just that; it is not a "child." Let your opponent and your audience know that a pregnant woman is not a "mother" unless she now has, or has had, a living child. Likewise a man who has impregnated a woman is not necessarily a "father"; he is more apt to be a sperm depositor. Remind them that abortion is not "murder"—it is a legal, medical procedure—and that slander and libel laws exist to protect persons unjustly accused of advocating murder.

Euphemisms are not honest, and there is no need to accept your opponent's estimate of him or herself as a "right-to-lifer." Those who oppose abortion are not "right-to-lifers," they are antiabortionists or compulsory-pregnancy people. Those who adhere to the pure Catholic doctrine, and do not believe in abortion even to save a

49

woman's life (and there are a surprising number of these on the speaking circuit), quite properly can be described as being against the right to life for women. Remind your audience that before abortion was legalized in the United States, many thousands of women were admitted every year to hospitals for care after botched abortions, and another 300 women died each year from backstreet or self-induced abortions.* Anyone wanting to return women to that situation does not respect life.

*If your opponent uses graphic aids, use yours, too.* If you are consenting to take the proabortion side of a discussion or debate, be sure you know the ground rules. If pictures, slides or films are being used by the opposition, get some of your own. If gory pictures are what is on the agenda, then go prepared with your own pictures of women dead from botched abortions, of deformed fetuses, beaten babies, and starving children.

Two short, informative films that are excellent aids in presentations are "Women Who've Lived Through Illegal Abortions" and "Aspiration Abortion."**

*Zero in on punitive attitudes.* If you have hostile people in your audience, questions will quite often have a punitive twist. Plan to pounce on them. The question quoted ear-lier: "If some sixteen-year-old tart goes out and gets her-

---

*The statistics game is a difficult one to play regarding abortion, because prior to its legality there were few firm figures available. In 1960, for example, 300 death certificates in the U.S. carried abortion as the cause of death, according to the Population Institute of New York City. However, because of the stigma attached to abortion and to out-of-wedlock pregnancy, it is logical to assume that many deaths from abortion went unreported as such, and were attributed to other causes, such as peritonitis. Data from the *National Health Survey* further indi-cate large numbers of illegal abortions reflected in hospital admissions, for women needing medical care as a result of interrupted pregnancies. Although these figures are not broken down and include spontaneous abortions, therapeutic abortions, and induced abortions, there were 358,000 such admissions in 1965, a figure that fell to 282,000 by 1971, when legal abortions were becoming regionally available.

**See Appendix D, "What You Can Do" for details.

self pregnant . . ." is a typical example of this—there's one like that in every audience. You will make points with your listeners when you note that a sixteen-year-old probably isn't a tart, that this may have been a first sexual experience or a forced sexual experience, that she obviously did not get herself pregnant, and that she needs an abortion, not the punishment of enforced pregnancy. "Why punish?" is a question I keep asking, and it is a question hostile people need to hear. Some religions bolster punitive attitudes in their followers. They preach tolerance, forgiveness, and understanding, but what comes through on the abortion issue is: "If she plays, she pays." Wanting people to be punished seems to be an old Christian habit.

*Don't be afraid to show emotion if you feel emotional.* It's warranted. Your opponent in most cases will be an individual who wants to deny abortion to any woman—to victims of rape, to child victims of incest, to women worn out from childbearing, to women who are ill, and even to women who may die if they are not aborted. Getting emotional in debates about tax structures may seem insincere; getting emotional about a woman's right to have an abortion is an inevitable reaction.

*Don't be apologetic.* Remember that no one has ever suggested a law compelling a woman to have an abortion. The premise you defend is that NO WOMAN SHOULD BE DENIED AN ABORTION BECAUSE OF THE RELIGIOUS BELIEFS OF OTHER PEOPLE.

# 8

# *Analyzing the Antis*

THE ANTIABORTIONISTS like to proclaim that theirs is an ecumenical movement, and not predominantly Catholic. Although statistics on the composition of their various groups are not public information, anyone who reads their literature, subscribes to their national newspaper, or attends one of their state or national gatherings cannot avoid the impression that Catholics are running the show. At one meeting of a Wisconsin group, the members spent an hour discussing whether they should identify themselves as Catholics in the letters they wrote to newspapers. Opinion was sharply divided on divulgence of this important information, not because there were non-Catholics present but because one faction thought it bad P.R. to be identified as Catholics, while the other argued that being Catholic is "nothing to be ashamed of."

Whether or not the Catholic composition of the antiabortion movement is in doubt, one fact is not, and that is that the resistance to giving women the right to choose abortion is *religious.* When you scan lists of groups opposing abortion, you find all of them are religious in nature.

Organized religion has done great harm to women. The pervading put-down of women detectable throughout the

Bible, the myth of Eve's sin, the ludicrousness of a virgin birth (as though there really were something wrong with ordinary sex)—all this has damaged women. Elizabeth Cady Stanton, who fought for women's equality in the nineteenth century, said forthrightly: "The Bible and the Church have been the greatest stumbling blocks in the way of women's emancipation." Another of her statements that has been widely quoted strikes a responsive chord with those exposed as children to dogmatic religions: "The memory of my own suffering has prevented me from ever shadowing one young soul with the superstitions of the Christian religion."

The desire of so many clergymen to keep women subservient, dependent, voiceless, is in itself an appalling commentary on both religion and male supremacy. Man has stood for so long with one foot on woman's neck that he finds he cannot stand up any other way. The posture is crippling.

Ostensibly we are a country devoted to the principle of separation of church and state, a principle that is germane to any discussion of abortion, because the conflict surrounding abortion is a conflict of the various beliefs on the beginning of life. There are obviously many beliefs about when life begins. Some people believe life starts at conception, others that life is present before conception and exists in the sperm and the egg. Some people believe life starts with movement of the fetus; the dictionary defines "quickening" as "to come alive." Others believe life starts with viability (capability of the fetus for independent survival). Still others think it starts with birth. One of the reasons abortion was so readily accepted by the Japanese was because the Shinto religion defines life as starting at birth.

Now, in a country which says church and state are separate, there should be room for all religious beliefs, particularly in areas of private concern where the public interest is not in question. The woman who believes life starts with conception should be free to carry through her pregnancy, just as the woman who believes life starts with quickening should be free to terminate her pregnancy.

But with no abortion laws, say opponents, women will be asking for abortions at eight and a half months. Not so. A woman who does not want to be pregnant does not want to stay pregnant a day longer than she has to. Women who want abortions want them early, the earlier the better. Many choose menstrual extraction when it is available, opting for the procedure even before a urine test to confirm their pregnancy is valid. Fewer and fewer women are seeking abortions after three months, as early abortion becomes more readily available to them. The longer the antiabortionists continue to fight legal abortion, the longer there will continue to be late abortions, because it is lack of access to abortion that results in late abortion in many cases. Almost the only women asking for second trimester (four to six month inclusive) abortions, in areas where abortion can be found easily, are teen-agers who have been afraid to tell anyone they are pregnant, women with highly irregular periods who have no way of knowing they are pregnant, or women who think they are in menopause and discover it is pregnancy. A surprising number of women have periods after becoming pregnant and find, to their dismay, that they are four or five months pregnant rather than the two or three months they had calculated. Women who suspect they are carrying damaged fetuses cannot receive confirmation of this through amniocentesis until the fourth month of pregnancy, and do not have the option of choosing early abortion.

\*     \*     \*

In Wisconsin the shrill insistence of the Catholic Church that all Wisconsin must live by Catholic doctrine is particularly ironic, when one realizes that Catholic women are the major group seeking abortions in Wisconsin. In 1971 in a survey of 200 consecutive women referred by Madison ZPG, 54 per cent were Catholic. Edith Rein, formerly of Milwaukee and the founder of the Wisconsin Committee to Legalize Abortion, the first referral group in the state,

55

reports 75 percent Catholic women referred over a four year period. Rev. Elinor Yeo of the Clergy Consultation Service in Milwaukee reports approximately 80 percent Catholic women referred in 1972 and 70 percent in 1973. The Catholic Church obviously cannot sell its ideas to its own people; what arrogance that it should attempt to impose these beliefs by law on others.

Instead of frantically attempting to bolster its fractured church by the same old pronouncements on the evils of contraception, sterilization, and abortion, the Catholic Church would be far more profitably and relevantly employed in asking itself: What have we done to our women? Why do so many Catholic women seek abortions?

The answers are obvious, of course. A woman brought up to regard contraception as sinful is far less apt to protect herself from an unwanted pregnancy than a woman who has been taught that contraception is intelligent. A Catholic woman is more apt to experiment with rhythm, one of the least effective methods of birth control. A Catholic woman is more apt to have been denied a tubal ligation by her Catholic physician in her Catholic hospital. She is more apt to seek abortion because she is worn out from childbearing, because she has had a baby every year until she is about to die from it.

Whenever I hear a Catholic priest condemning abortion, I remember the young woman whom I counseled extensively both before and after her abortion, who needed far more support than most of the women I refer. She had been impregnated by her priest.

The most unsuccessful birth control and abortion reform groups in this country have been led by those who say, "But what will people think if we criticize religion? We don't want to alienate our Catholic friends." It's a cop-out and a very serious one. When I first heard that the pro-abortion forces working to win the referendum in Michigan were not planning to utilize religious arguments in their battle, and were going to refrain scrupulously from any criticism of the Catholic Church, I shuddered. This is what the battle is all about. When the Catholic Church is trying to ram its doctrine down the throats of everyone in sight, you are not going to beat them off if you tiptoe around saying how nice they are.

The progress that has been brought about in women's rights, and birth control and abortion law reform, has been brought about *despite* the Catholic Church, not because of it. There is no point in our pretending that official Catholic views are enlightened and humane, or that Catholics are not different from anyone else. Catholics are different from others—they are quite willing to associate themselves with an organization that has done and continues to do an immense amount of damage to women, to families, to countries, and to the world. If the Catholic doctrines on sex (no contraception, no sterilization, no abortion) could prevail, all the world would be miserable instead of just some of it. All the world would be hungry. The world would end.

Repeatedly in my conversations with Catholics around the state of Wisconsin, I have urged those who have expressed sympathy with the contraception and abortion causes to start a "Catholics for the Right to Choose Abortion" or "Fond du Lac Catholics for Contraceptive Law Repeal." To a woman (or man), they have shuffled their feet, looked uncomfortable, and said, "Oh, I couldn't do that." When I say, "Well, at least quit giving money to your church and tell your priest why—no more money until these positions are changed," they reply, "Oh, but our priest is quite liberal." People like this are part of the problem; they are not part of the solution. They are totally unwilling to accept responsibility for the monstrous actions of their church.

If people had chosen to tiptoe around other harmful organizations, for example the Ku Klux Klan, and say, "Oh, they mean well; they're really nice people," the Klan would prosper. It is social disapproval and social pressure, as well as intellectual persuasion, that causes individuals to avoid groups or stop supporting them. If, through politeness, we smile and agree with our Catholic acquaintances that there are indeed many liberal Catholic priests, and, yes, hasn't the Church changed, they are going to keep on forking out the money and support that keeps the Catholic Church going, and buttresses its continued denial to women *all over the world* their right to practice contraception and have sterilizations and abortions.

Think of the millions of dollars the antiabortionists have already spent attempting to deny American women their right to choose abortion. Financial support for antiabortion candidates, full page ads in the country's most expensive newspapers, demonstrations, radio and television ads, books placed in libraries, films and slide shows, their own antiabortion newspaper—think of the *good* that money might have done. All over the world there are miserable, starving, needy Catholic children. Why, in the name of morality, aren't they helping children already born, rather than trying to force unwilling women to produce more unwanted children?

Think of the "Birthright" groups, those antiabortion counseling services that follow the lead of their mentors, the so-called "Right-to-Lifers." They, too, like to emphasize that they are not really Catholic groups, but ecumenical groups, and that is is sheer coincidence that so many of their offices are located on the premises of Catholic welfare organizations, such as homes for unwed mothers.

Another coincidence seems to be that Birthright, like the Catholic Church, opposes contraception and sterilization as well as abortion. Article III, Section 2 of the Birthright Charter Document reads:

> The Policy of every Birthright Chapter and everyone of its members and volunteers is all that chapter's efforts shall be to refrain in every instance from offering or giving advice on the subjects of contraception or sterilization, and to refrain from referring any person to another person, place or agency for this type of service.

58

No contraception, no sterilizations, no abortions—tell us, Birthright, what are women supposed to do?

But the real pity of the Birthright movement lies not in its attempts to conceal its Catholic pedigree, but in its conception as an antiabortion gesture—not out of concern for women, but because of adherence to religious doctrine. Had there been no freedom for women to choose abortion, there would have been no Birthright movement. The frightened pregnant woman who needed someone to turn to was always there. Birthright materialized and took an interest in her only when her right to choose abortion challenged sectarian belief.

Along about my two hundredth abortion referral, I became aware of a sort of refrain among the callers. "I asked my doctor for the pill, but he is Catholic and he won't help me." "I wanted a tubal ligation, but my doctor is Catholic and he wouldn't do it." "The specialist said not to have another baby or I might not live through it, but our hospital here is Catholic, and he couldn't do a ligation." Or, "After my last baby I wanted to go on the pill, but we're Catholic, and my husband wouldn't let me."

There is no way of assembling and evaluating the damage done to women, families, and society by the Catholic Church, but we can talk about it. Not to do so would be the equivalent of the emancipators of 120 years ago saying, "Oh, they own slaves, but they're nice people, so we won't say anything."

Birth control and abortion are our greatest steps forward in social and moral progress since we freed the slaves. A woman's right to control her own reproductive life is a blessing, a blessing for her and a blessing for society. There is no reason to be bashful or apologetic about supporting women's freedom to choose abortion; there is every reason to be ashamed of supporting a religion that opposes that freedom.

# 9

# *What Can We Do About Medicine?*

WOMEN, THOSE SECOND-CLASS CITIZENS, have suffered long and silently from an elitist medical profession dominated by males. When a general practitioner or a gynecologist goes out to a small community and will not, as many in Wisconsin still do not, offer birth control, sterilization, or abortions to his patients, the state is allowing the medical profession to place individual religious views above the health and welfare of its citizens. When women with four and five Caesarean sections are denied tubal ligations by their physicians, a familiar story in Wisconsin, we might as well be licensing Jack the Ripper or Richard Speck. Because women are going to suffer and women are going to die.

From 1969 to 1971 in Wisconsin forty-eight women died in pregnancy, thirty-two of whom had serious and compelling medical reasons not to be pregnant at all.* Unbelievably these victims included a woman whose scar from a classical Caesarean section had ruptured in her last pregnancy. What did these medical boobs think would happen, allowing her to become and remain pregnant again? One

*Herbert Sandmire, M.D., "Family Planning Comes of Age?" *Wisconsin Medical Journal,* April, 1972, pp. 71-72.

woman who had had seven pregnancies, and suffered from hypertension of several years duration, requested an abortion, which was denied. One day prior to her own death, she delivered a stillborn, macerated fetus. No doubt her doctor still is allowed to practice his lethal brand of medicine and her hospital still is receiving public funds!

Other women in this Wisconsin study, who died from pregnancy, had diabetes, breast cancer, heart disease or disorders, histories of toxemia and hypertension, four and five previous Caesarean sections. They might as well have lived in remotest Upper Slobovia, for in far too many communities in Wisconsin a woman's life and health still do not matter—what matters is the religion of her physician and of those who control the local hospital.

In Wisconsin there are 145 hospitals for short-term patient care in the state. Of these 133 are classed as "private." In many communities the only obstetrical services available are from Catholic-owned or dominated hospitals. What are women to do under this sort of medical dictatorship? And is there such a thing any more as a "private" hospital? All hospitals receive huge infusions of the public's money, and they should be operated by medical, not religious standards. A state government does not license doctors or hospitals for *their* benefit, but for the public's benefit. When will the idea of *service* penetrate that armor of insensitivity surrounding the medical community?

A new wrinkle in hospital practice in cities having two or three hospitals is the channeling of maternity patients to one facility. All too often the facility chosen is a Catholic hospital, and women needing sterilizations at the time of delivery find their medical needs ignored because of religious prejudice. Neonatal units (for high risk newborns), serving wide geographic areas, are occasionally located in Catholic hospitals, and the pregnant woman again is in a captive situation. Sterilizations are sought more often by women after high-risk pregnancies, and these patients' serious medical needs again are shunted aside. Catholic hospitals delight in proclaiming their moral objections to abortion, yet every time they deny a woman a sterilization they have created a candidate for abortion.

In the backlash of the United States Supreme Court decision on abortion, Congress and many states have passed laws specifying that any hospital, public or private, may turn away any woman for sterilization or abortion, no matter what her physical condition, even if she has a doctor willing to help her. These laws have been challenged successfully insofar as public hospitals are concerned, but, unbelievably, the private hospital exemption has been allowed to stand. While such laws have limited effect in large, urban communities with a choice of hospitals for women and doctors, they seriously jeopardize freedom of choice and humane health care for women who have one local hospital.

These laws, of course, discriminate against women, since men do not need abortions and can have their sterilizations performed in doctor's offices. Women need a hospital for a second trimester abortion and for a sterilization. Such laws discriminate against the poor. If a well-to-do woman is denied an abortion or tubal ligation in her own community, she has the money and resources to seek these services elsewhere. But if the poor woman is not served by her local community, she is rarely served at all.

No hospital should be allowed to deny emergency treatment to women. When a woman is having a fourth or fifth Caesarean section, she needs a tubal ligation; this *is* an emergency situation. When a woman becomes pregnant, who has diabetes or hypertension or a heart disorder or any of a dozen other serious conditions, she needs an abortion; these are emergency situations. Too many women suffer and die because hospital policy ranks higher with male physicians, male legislators, and male judges than women's lives and health.

In 1974, 5,000 applicants, many of them women, applied for 121 medical school openings at the Wisconsin Medical College in Milwaukee.* While some of these applicants were accepted at other schools, and many did not

*Milwaukee Journal, Sept. 8, 1974

have the necessary academic qualifications, there were still large numbers of qualified would-be physicians who were turned away. Here we are, the richest country in the world, and qualified women and men who wish to become doctors may not do so because we do not have the capacity to train them. The most important single thing we can do to improve health care in our country is to train more doctors, and to be sure that at least half of them are women, and that blacks and other minorities are represented fairly. Who knows—with enough doctors to help, maybe house calls might be fashionable again?*

In addition to training more doctors we must check the screening procedures used in acceptance of applicants. Medical schools must not look just for academic excellence, but for social concern, some evidence of social commitment, some awareness in the applicant of the dignity and worth of all people. Too often a physician comes across not as a patient advocate, but as a patient adversary. The qualities of consideration and warmth are ignored. One cannot avoid the impression that most medical schools in the past have screened for political conservatives.

Since a medical education is the most expensive education we offer, and since the medical student pays for only a small portion of that education (15 percent at the University of Wisconsin, Madison), it is fair and proper that we expect certain things of these privileged persons. If a stu-

---

* In 1955 I had had twin babies via Caesarean section (a third Caesarean), with my medical history further embellished by a ruptured appendix earlier in that pregnancy. I was nursing the babies, having an abundance of milk, but developed a breast infection when they were about a month old. I was really very sick, with chills and raging fever. The doctor diagnosed and prescribed over the phone. When a couple of days passed and my fever still raged, the doctor suggested that I come in for an office visit. I explained what he must have known—that I was too weak to do that, that my fever edged up a notch or two just getting up to go to the bathroom. When I recovered and went in a week or so later to be checked, he said, "Well, we got through that one all right, didn't we?" I would agree that the patient going to the doctor makes sense most of the time, but there are occasions when house calls are warranted, even for obstetricians.

64

dent wishes to become a gynecologist or obstetrician, the student should understand that she/he will be expected to help women with birth control and do tubal ligations and abortions. Medical students must be screened, and if they possess convictions that prevent their delivering certain medical care, then they should either specialize in an area where they cannot damage their patients with their personal beliefs, or perhaps they should consider the church, not medicine.

In addition, since this is such an expensive education that we provide, there is no reason why we should not ask these women and men, who have been chosen for this coveted training, to serve in areas without doctors for two years, or perhaps a period equivalent to their academic training? Who knows—they might like the communities that need them, and when they wished to leave, new graduates would be coming along. This is a practical, feasible answer to the distribution problem.

If we had a shortage of persons wanting and qualified to be physicians, we would have some excuse for being in the bind we are in. We do not have that shortage. Our problem is one of priorities, and our priorities can be changed!

The letter that follows is just an "every day" letter that illustrates the problems caused by doctors imposing religious views on their patients. This young couple had decided to opt for permanent birth control but could find no doctor to help them.


Dear ZPG:

I wrote to you about eight months ago. My husband wanted a vasectomy and you were very good to give us a list of doctors from this area who perform this surgery. We contacted the doctors but no one would do it because my husband is only twenty-four.

At that time I had tried the pill and had very bad reactions, and the doctor did not want to give it to me. So they put in an IUD that worked for one year, and now I am pregnant.

We have prepared ourselves for a baby, knowing we will try to make good parents. But the point is that after four years of marriage and two years of going together, we had definitely decided we did not want children. Now with one baby coming we are already worrying about what method of birth control we can use next.

We can't understand why this decision should not be ours. We are old enough to vote and pay taxes and run a business of our own, but we aren't old enough to decide if we want a family or not. We have discussed all the angles many times and this is still our choice.

So if there is anything you can do to help us now we would appreciate it. Thank you.     R.S.

The medical community could do so many painless things to improve its image and its services. Boards of Medical Examiners, for instance, should not all be physicians; they should have consumer representation. Medical societies should offer referrals. There should be a place to call and find out where one can get, for example, a safe tonsillectomy at the lowest cost. There should be simple procedures for registering complaints about treatment and charges.

Recently I referred a woman for abortion, who had a three-year-old child and an eleven-week-old baby. She said her doctor, a specialist, had told her as long as she was nursing and used foam, she would not get pregnant. She believed him, and she got pregnant. Now, you could forgive a doctor like that if he were some old, overworked, country GP, but a specialist! Doesn't he read the literature? She could have got advice as sound from any occult. And here she is—she doesn't want to have an abortion, but what is she to do?

Besides giving out a great deal of misinformation and

incomplete information on contraception, many doctors will not tell women of the risks involved in closely spaced pregnancies, or the risks of childbirth. Some of them love to represent abortion as involving risk, but they will not tell women that delivery involves greater risk. A careful specialist will see that his patient goes off the pill every two to three years for a few months time, to let her ovaries work on their own, but there are specialists who will never let on to their patients that four, five or even seven straight years on the pill is a risk they should not take.

Personal action is certainly in order for every woman in this country concerned with women's medical care. First of all, quiz *your* doctor. If he is opposed to contraception, sterilization, or abortion, dump him. Even if it means the inconvenience of going to another community, don't patronize him. If you are lucky and he is not a sexist, that is still no reason to be in awe of him. If he goofs, let him know. If his charges are excessive, complain. He has had a privileged education, tax-supported for the most part. He should be serving patients, not running his own private dictatorship.

Over the past few years my own attitude toward the medical profession has undergone a rather painful metamorphosis. I summed it up in a speech before a medical group in the spring of 1971, the chapter that follows.

# 10

# *Why Are You All So Angry?*

MOST OF MY LIFE I have been somewhat in awe of doctors. I have shared the general view that the profession was noble and the practitioners worthy of respect. My deference was so pronounced that my husband used to tease me, saying I failed to get my money's worth out of trips to the doctor. I was habitually reluctant to discuss my aches and pains to any degree when I actually was in the doctors' offices, because my symptoms seemed so trivial in light of the serious cases I knew they had to treat. And I appreciated that they must frequently be tired, probably overworked, at least pressed for time. I was pleased to have doctors as business friends and acquaintances, and I shared the traditional admiring attitude elicited by a physician's presence in any gathering.

But now all that has changed. I am a pronounced critic of the medical profession. I am on speaking terms only with two or three of my former medical friends and acquaintances. I no longer read or respect the *AMA News*. We even boo at our house when Marcus Welby comes on TV.

The reason? In my work for abortion reform I have learned that most doctors care more for their bank balances, their colleagues' opinions, their comfortable, unjeopardized way of life than they do for the health and welfare of their women patients.

When a federal court declared last March that the Wisconsin abortion law was unconstitutional and that the state of Wisconsin could no longer deprive a woman of her right to terminate an early, unwanted pregnancy, I was elated. Now, I thought, the doctors will help these women. Yet in the whole state of Wisconsin with its thousands of doctors, only one acted—Dr. Alfred Kennan of the University of Wisconsin Medical School. Calls came pouring into University Hospital from all over the country—as many as seventy in a day, with special-delivery letters and wires adding to that count. The hospital administration very quickly adopted a quota, understandable since they are a training hospital, but totally unrealistic in that only about five to eight abortions weekly were to be performed.

Because of my work with the Wisconsin Committee to Legalize Abortion my own phone started to ring, and I was able to get a few of these patients requesting abortions into University Hospital. But what to do with the others? I phoned every gynecologist in Madison asking for his help. Few were even polite to me. Only one showed any compunction about turning down my request. At the time I phoned one of the patients I specifically was trying to help was a fifteen-year-old girl from a broken home, whose very young age and tragic family situation I thought would surely elicit sympathy. Not a chance! I turned next on behalf of this girl to Milwaukee specialists. One doctor made an appointment and on the day of the appointment cancelled it. Another saw her after a ten-day wait and then refused to do the abortion. The search had been time consuming and by this time the girl had passed the deadline for the D & C. Since my only other safe source at this time was in Mexico City and because it seemed impossible to have a fifteen-year-old go that far away alone, I kept phoning Milwaukee doctors and finally found a crusader who did accept her. However, the salting out did not progress well, there were complications and she was in serious condition for two days before recovery. My relief to have her well and happy again was somewhat tempered by the fact that her hospital bill was in excess of $1,000, and by my knowledge that if there had been one Madison doctor who cared about a teen-aged girl's right *not* to become a mother, she could have had a safe, simple, inexpensive abortion in early pregnancy.

About this time two or three Madison organizations interested in abortion reform arranged a meeting with Madison General Hospital, a community-supported facility. Women's Liberation people spoke on the side of abortion; a pediatrician, a psychologist and a Unitarian clergyman from my committee urged the hospital to perform abortions. But the doctors from the hospital and its administrators told us they had no intention of doing abortions. It was one of the low points of my life as I listened to male after male speak against having the hospital offer this service. The final straw was the chief of staff who took the podium and talked about his "reverence for life." The meeting broke up into informal arguments and as I left the room I heard one doctor dramatically exclaim, "Why are you all so angry?"

I had not been asked to speak that night and the doctor's rhetorical question went unanswered, but I have often thought of what that answer should have been.

We are angry because for the first time we have seen the need for abortion that you must have seen throughout your careers and would do nothing about. We are angry because the court has given you the opportunity to help women who do not want to be pregnant, yet you will not take that opportunity, even though it brings you much money and much gratitude.

We are angry because we have seen and heard so much tragedy, so much avoidable tragedy. We cannot understand why you would want a fifteen-year-old girl who is physically immature, mentally immature, desperately unhappy, her education incomplete, to become a mother,

71

when you possess the skill and have the legal right to help her.

We are angry because we think of the women throughout human history who have had to endure unwanted pregnancies. We know, now, at this time, women who are too poor to have another baby, who have too many children already. We know women who have begged their doctors for contraceptives or for tubal ligations, and who are now pregnant because they were refused. How, we wonder, do you have the audacity to turn away the woman who wants an abortion when you would not help her prevent that pregnancy?

We know, as we are sure you know too, how many victims of incest and rape there really are in Wisconsin. How, we ask, can you be so inhumane as to turn away a thirteen-year-old girl and her eleven-year-old sister, who have been impregnated by their mother's "boy friend"?

And what about those pregnant girls who cry throughout conversations with you because their boy friends have gone—gone to California, or gone to Florida, or "We were to be married, but I don't know where he is now"?

What about the mother who has had a baby every year? Can't you recognize that a pregnant woman with five little children, the youngest three months, has a legitimate claim to any doctor's help and sympathy?

You ask why we are all so angry. We answer with a question. How can you be so cruel?

# 11

# *Every Five Days*
# *There Are One Million*
# *More Of Us*

THE STARVING CHILDREN have come into our living rooms
now. There they are on the network evening news lining
up for a cup of milk, or bony hands outstretched, jostling
for a bit of food. We were told this would happen. Back in
1950 scholars were predicting this. But ours was the country of surpluses and it was not a problem of scarcity, most
said, but a problem of distribution. In 1950 poor India
appealed to the World Health Organization (WHO) for
help with contraception, but the Catholic member nations
of WHO made their usual outcry, and what India got in
1950, when the problem still might have been alleviated,
was a team of experts to teach—you guessed it: *rhythm!*

Now the signs of disaster are everywhere. Food shortages, fuel shortages, fertilizer shortages, unemployment,
pollution, dust bowls, encroaching deserts, disease. For
it is a truth that population is going to be controlled. If
it is not controlled by women's and men's intellect, it will
be controlled by famine, disease, and war.

Sharing the American continent are countries so poor
that most of their people are malnourished, yet these
countries will double their populations in the next twenty

73

years. The question is inescapable: when these governments cannot take care of the people they have now, how can they be expected to keep up with the demands of ever-burgeoning populations?

How long will our neighbors to the south allow each other to live in peace? How long will the United States and Canada remain islands of affluence while the rest of the hemisphere suffers? What would you do if it were your kids that were hungry?

Food is only one problem—health and education are critical problems, too. In all the six central American countries there are fewer physicians than we have in the state of Tennessee, and Tennessee is not known for its advanced health care. In El Salvador for every one hundred students in the first grade in 1967, eighty failed to graduate from the sixth grade, and untold numbers never find their way to school at all.* Health care should be the right of every child in the world and how do you break the poverty cycle without education, without some preparation for jobs?

We live today on a crowded and polluted planet where population control has become our single most important problem. Every five days there are one million more persons on earth. Even with the much-heralded dip in the United States birthrate, our own country added almost 1.5 million persons to its numbers last year, some through immigration, but most through added births. The reality of overpopulation confronts almost every country, yet in much of the world contraception remains limited, sterilization unavailable, and abortion illegal.

---

*C. Capa, and J. M. Stycos, *Margin of Life* (New York: Grossman Publishers, 1974), p. 6.

# 12

# Do We Belong
# in The Kitchen?

PREGNANCY IS NOT something you do; it is something that happens to you.

Far too often pregnancy has been compulsory, and its limited emergence as an elective already is shaking society. That the women's liberation movement in America coexists with a drop in the birthrate is not coincidence. True equality for all women will have as its immediate by-product a drop in the number of births. Real freedom to control reproduction will change the world because women never wanted all those babies—they had them because they couldn't help it.

When most cultures regard women as breeding machines, and most of the world does just that, of course populations will grow. When you are brought up not to please yourself, but to please men, naturally you are going to breed. Left to be free you might use your creativity to be a composer or inventor or architect, but if the role that is forced on you is that of wife and mother, you must be very strong indeed to overthrow tradition. When in school you are steered toward home economics or typing, and to become a cheerleader is the begin-all, end-all of existence, of course you are going to turn out to be a breeder. If cheering on the men rather than achieving things yourself is what you are judged by, then quite naturally you will fall into the pregnancy trap.

In the United States we are taking the first steps toward a society that will see women as persons, not sex objects. We are moving toward a society that will give women equal opportunities in the professions and trades, where the criterion for employment will be ability, not sex. Such a society will produce happier women and men. Such a society will produce fewer children, but such children will be treasured because they will not be accidents, or duties, or someone else's expectations—they will be wanted children.

Feminist and author Elizabeth Janeway, who always has something thoughtful to say, addressed the annual meeting of the National Abortion Rights Action League (NARAL) in Washington D.C. in October, 1973. Commenting on the possibility of the United States Supreme Court decision on abortion being overthrown, Ms Janeway concluded: "If we lose this one, we belong in the kitchen."

But we're not going to lose this one. Male supremacists, fundamentalists, and the Catholic Church finally have met their match. Feminists will work until the freedom to choose abortion is extended to women everywhere. Women no longer belong in the kitchen. They belong, as equal persons, in the world.

# 13

# "Why Don't They Just Use Birth Control?"

WHENEVER I SPEAK ON ABORTION an inevitable question is: "Why don't women just use birth control?"

It is my own experience in referring women for abortions that about 38 percent of them *are practicing birth control* at the time they become pregnant. Some of the methods being used are most unreliable—foam, rhythm, withdrawal, but people are trying. Out of each hundred women I refer, I can count on three or four of them having IUD's in place. Although most IUD failures seem to occur in the first year of use, I have referred a woman for abortion whose IUD had worked for her for *nine* years. Women getting pregnant with them after two or three years of successful use is not at all unusual. The Dalkon shield, the crab-shaped IUD so popular with physicians, is the most unreliable of the well-known IUD's. Recently it was withdrawn from the market, since it apparently was the cause of serious uterine infections, some fatal, in women who became pregnant while it was in place.

The pill, of course, is an effective method of birth control, but even with its good record of reliability some women still get pregnant on it—they do not forget to take it—there are occasional legitimate pill failures. One woman I referred for abortion became pregnant twice on the pill. The first time she carried her pregnancy to term, and then her doctor prescribed a stronger pill. She took it faithfully and she took it at the same time every day just to be very sure. And she conceived a second time, even on a high estrogen-content pill.

Although pill failures are relatively rare, serious reactions to the pill are common. Many women who have family histories of blood-clotting diseases should not take it at all. Women subject to migraine headaches, asthma, varicose veins or high blood pressure may worsen their conditions on it. Liver disease, kidney disease, diabetes, epilepsy, heart disease or defect, and cancer usually preclude use of the pill.

For many women the decision to take the pill is out of their hands because it makes them so sick—there is no question of their continuing on it. Unhappily many women stay on the pill despite side effects because their contraception options are so limited.

In addition to being so imperfect, contraception is still unavailable, especially to young people and to poor people. Many states still have laws restricting the visibility and accessibility of contraceptives. For instance in Wisconsin condoms legally may not be sold in machines, and crusader Bill Baird was arrested in 1971 for displaying "indecent articles" in a public lecture. Until a federal court ruling in November, 1974, unmarried persons in Wisconsin legally could not use contraceptives. As long as contraception remains as imperfect as it is and as unavailable as it is, we can expect women to resort to abortion.

Those who ask, "Why don't they just use birth control?" must be reminded that sex education is trivial or nonexistent in many schools. The student learns in the typical biology or health class that sex may result in pregnancy, but she/he is not told how to avoid that pregnancy. In addition, many Catholic women and men are brought up to believe that contraception is sinful, and consequently they take chances they would not take had this particular indoctrination not befallen them.

78

Getting pregnant is very easy. Educating people how not to get pregnant is a gargantuan task, especially in a state like Wisconsin, which has an anticontraceptive law uniquely constructed to make dissemination of information as difficult as possible.

Two very common causes of birth-control failure are dependence on a so-called "safe period," and using condoms for ejaculation only.

I am not a fan of billboards, but I would like to see a few on every major highway across the country saying, "There is no such thing as a safe period." Although most women are apt to conceive midway between periods, I have referred women for abortions whose only intercourse was just before a menstrual period, just after a menstrual period, even during a menstrual period. It is a fact that ovaries can release eggs any old time. The only way for someone to be reasonably sure she does not conceive is to use an effective method of birth control *all the time*.

Packages of condoms should carry instructions in big, bold print that this product must be used *throughout* intercourse if it is to be an effective method of birth control. Too often men do not use condoms throughout sex, but only for ejaculation. Sperms escape prior to ejaculation, and pregnancy results.

All of our present methods of birth control are very poor; all have serious shortcomings. The pill's chief liability is its unpleasant, sometimes dangerous side effects; the IUD its pain in insertion, the cramping and heavy menstrual flow it frequently causes, and its unreliability for many women. Foam, of course, is grossly unreliable, and despite what the ads say should never be used alone, only with condoms or a diaphragm. Condoms interfere with touch; many women have aesthetic objections to diaphragms or worry that they may slip out of position. So there you are. It's too bad some of the money we have spent on munitions could not have been spent on research for contraceptives.

When someone says to me, "Why don't women just use birth control?" I am reminded of the member of Birthright who called me long distance for abortion referral information. She was very distraught, half-crying and said, "I always thought of myself as helping these young girls. I never thought of women like me getting pregnant." Her method of birth control had always worked for her, and she was devastated when it failed.

When some woman shakes her head and says, "I could *never* have an abortion," through my mind pass the dozens and dozens of conversations I have had that started out with the caller saying, "I never dreamed I would be calling a service like yours . . . I never believed in abortion . . . I never thought I would want an abortion, but . . ."

Never is a long, long time.

14

# Late Abortion
# and The Edelin Case

WHEN DR. KENNETH EDELIN was found guilty of manslaughter by a Boston jury in February, 1975, in the
alleged death of a fetus following a legal abortion, the
story broke on a Saturday afternoon, and we in Madison
braced ourselves for the interpretive reporting of the *Wis-*
*consin State Journal,* Madison's conservative morning newspaper. Sure enough! There in a type size appropriate for
the announcement of World War III was the antiabortion
version of what had happened. "ABORTION RULED A
KILLING" exulted Sunday morning's banner headline.

That gentle Dr. Edelin ever should have found himself a
defendant against a charge of manslaughter beggars
belief. Reared in a black district of Washington D.C., he
attended segregated schools there. One of four children,
three of whom went to college, he graduated from Colum-
bia University in New York in 1961, taught math and
science for awhile, and then decided to take up medicine,
graduating from Meharry Medical College in Nashville.

He became the first black chief resident of obstetrics-
gynecology in the history of Boston City Hospital, a hospital which serves a largely black clientele. After the historic

Supreme Court decision legalizing abortion in 1973, he performed abortions at the hospital for the women who requested them.

In October, 1973, a black woman brought her seventeen-year-old unmarried daughter to Dr. Edelin for an abortion. Estimating her pregnancy at approximately twenty-one to twenty-two weeks, Dr. Edelin proceeded with the saline-injection method of abortion, which usually causes uterine contractions and expulsion of the fetus. When attempts at repeated saline injections were unsuccessful, he performed the abortion surgically by a procedure called hysterotomy, a miniature Caesarean section. His patient had a normal recovery.

Prior to this time in Boston, four scientists, all medical doctors, were trying to find alternate drugs to prescribe for pregnant women allergic to penicillin. They had studied, with the consent of the patients involved, thirty-three women who were having abortions. Two antibiotic drugs, clindamycin and erythromycin, were given the women prior to their abortions, and the aborted fetuses were then studied, to see which drug more readily passed the placental barrier. Their findings, that clindamycin passes through more easily than erythromycin, and that either drug is a reasonable alternative to penicillin in the treatment of intrauterine infections, were published in the *New England Journal of Medicine.** Antiabortionists, to whom fetal research is anathema even though it is conducted to help women retain pregnancies, called this article to the attention of Massachusetts State Representative Raymond Flynn, who took the issue to a Boston City Council member, Albert O'Neill, who in turn called it to the attention of Boston District Attorney Garrett Byrne.**** In Byrne's ensuing investigation, the twenty-one to twenty-two week

*Agneta Philipson, M.D., L.D. Sabath, M.D., and David Charles, M.D., "Transplacental Passage of Erythromycin and Clindamycin," *New England Journal of Medicine,* (June 7, 1973).
**Boston Globe, (Jan. 5, 1975). Subsequent direct quotations in this chapter, unless otherwise attributed, come from the *Boston Globe,* (Jan. 5, 12, 19, Feb. 16, 17, 1975).

fetus Dr. Edelin had aborted was discovered at the mortuary by the antiabortionists. Grand jury proceedings followed. Eventually, unbelievably, the four doctors engaged in fetal experimentation were charged under a nineteenth century "grave-robbing" statute (case pending), and Dr. Edelin was charged with manslaughter. Alice-in-Wonderland never knew what she missed by not visiting Boston.

The six-weeks trial of Dr. Edelin, a trial that never should have taken place, attracted nationwide attention. The prosecutor, forty-four-year-old Assistant District Attorney Newman A. Flanagan, was described repeatedly by the *Boston Globe* in flattering terms. "His reputation for wit and flair matches his record as a tough prosecutor," trilled the *Globe*. Examples of his wit were recorded: he explained his gray hair as a result of "early piety" and "he might pick up a dead phone and say for the amusement of his fellow prosecutors 'Tell Cronkite I'm too busy . . . No, no, I haven't got time to be interviewed by *Newsweek*.'"
That he was the father of seven children was duly reported by the Boston paper, along with his eldest son's athletic prowess. The full roster of prosecutors' names—Flanagan, Mulligan, Brennan and Dunn—sounded like roll call at an Irish wake.

Judge for the trial in Suffolk's Superior Court was James McGuire, a graduate of Catholic University and Boston University School of Law. The *Boston Globe* cited his "reputation for competency" and for "keeping lawyers from straying off the central issue."

This "reputation for competency" was put to an early test. William Homans, the attorney for Dr. Edelin, asked to have the case thrown out of court on the basis of the jury pool. In Boston, a "sexist" computer chooses names of prospective jurors; it is programmed to put out two men's names for every one woman's name. In addition, the registrar is instructed to mail out the summons for jury duty on a two-to-one, male-preferred basis. This blatant discrimination against women did not move Judge McGuire, who denied Homans' request. The all-white jury that was selected was predominantly male; only three women were chosen. Ten of the twelve persons finally deciding Dr. Edelin's fate were Catholic.

That card-carrying, dues-paying Catholics ever should have been allowed to serve on a jury deciding a charge of abortion-related manslaughter is a travesty of justice. They support the institution that is the major enemy of abortion in the world—yet they were allowed to bring their religious bias to this legal setting.

Examination of jurors is extremely restrictive in Massachusetts. It is all done by the judge alone. Although the defense attorneys and the prosecution may submit questions for the judge to ask, there is no delving permitted and a very limited number of challenges allowed. In a case as serious as Edelin's, lawyers for the defendant are understandably reluctant to use up all their challenges early in the jury screening, since far more biased potential jurors could be expected to be coming down the pike.

The prosecution stumbled early in its case, when one of its major witnesses against Dr. Edelin testified that she had not been in the operating room at all at the time the hysterotomy took place. In essence, the only witness against Dr. Edelin turned out to be Dr. Enrique Gimenez-Jimeno, who testified that Dr. Edelin, after detaching the placenta from the uterine wall, held the fetus within the woman's uterus for three minutes while looking at a clock on the operating room wall. Such an action would deprive a fetus of oxygen. Gimenez-Jimeno's testimony was refuted by all other eye-witnesses, who stated that the hysterotomy took place with no unusual delays and that the clock Dr. Gimenez referred to was not there at all, as it had been taken out for repairs.

"Experts," whose qualifications included leadership positions in the antiabortion movement, told the jurors that in their opinion the fetus was viable despite its early gestational age. Other witnesses testified that in their judgment the fetus was nonviable, that it not only never breathed, but was incapable of breathing. Dr. Edelin told the jury that he would not perform an abortion if he

84

believed the fetus might live independently from the woman.

"I have never performed an abortion on a woman who was carrying a fetus I considered to be viable," Dr. Edelin testified. "In fact, I have refused to perform such abortions."

At the close of the trial the names of the sixteen jurors were placed in a small metal drum and four slips were removed. These four, who became the alternate jurors and did not participate in the verdict, ironically turned out to be the two youngest and the two most educated members of the panel.

"We polled ourselves," said Michael Ciano, one of the four, "and three of us voted for Dr. Edelin's acquittal."

The other twelve jurors retired to discuss the case, and did not reach a verdict for seven hours. The defense had been hopeful when Judge McGuire charged the jury, because he instructed them that manslaughter required the death of a person, which was defined as an infant born alive and able to exist outside the uterus. Dr. Edelin said later his own optimism dimmed as the first day of deliberation passed and no verdict was reached. When the jury recessed for the night on Friday, he was worried. Shortly after one o'clock on Saturday afternoon, Feb. 15, 1975, the jury brought in its verdict. Foreman Vincent Shea forcefully called out their finding: "Guilty."

Dr. Edelin said he saw the guilty verdict on the faces of the jurors even before the foreman shouted it.

"When the jury came in not one of them would look me in the eye," he said. "I became very apprehensive. As it turned out the die was cast when we picked the jurors. . . . It was a witch-hunt. I don't think the jury was fair. I don't think it would have been possible to get a fair jury in Suffolk County, no matter how many challenges we might have had."

Later certain jury members were to say that a photograph of the fetus shown to them by Prosecutor Flanagan decided them in their finding of Dr. Edelin's guilt, because "it looked like a baby." Since there was no question of the legality of the abortion procedure, the jurors had to be convinced beyond a reasonable doubt that Dr. Edelin had been guilty of negligence following the abortion. A photograph of a preserved fetus scarcely gives credence to a charge of negligence. It is probably the first time in courtroom history that a defendant was found guilty because his alleged victim looked like a person!

Racial bias may have abetted religious bias, according to alternate juror Michael Ciano, who charged that racial slurs against Dr. Edelin had been made more than once before closing arguments. Although other jurors were to deny this, Ciano quoted one juror as saying, "That black nigger is as guilty as sin."

Dr. Edelin remained outwardly composed after the verdict, but others in the courtroom did not. There were sobs and cries of disbelief as spectators said to each other, "How could they find him guilty?" Several women left the courtroom looking dazed and stunned; some were crying openly. Those who had followed the testimony day after day were especially disbelieving.

"Edelin's attorneys countered the philosophical arguments and they countered the factual arguments," one feminist told me. "The overwhelming weight of evidence was on our side. When the mainstay of the testimony against Dr. Edelin is the word of one man, who reportedly held personal animosity toward him and who based his testimony on a clock that wasn't even there—well, that jury was just dumb."

That Judge McGuire may have shared her opinion seems a likely speculation. According to a report in the *Globe*, he, too, seemed "stunned" by the verdict, and did not thank the jury as is customary after a long trial. Three days later he sentenced Dr. Edelin to one year's probation.

The Edelin case is being appealed to the Supreme Judicial Court of Massachusetts, with oral arguments probably being heard in the fall of 1975. Although there can be little question that the conviction will be overturned, and that the final fallout from the trial will be favorable, its immediate effect was that many of the doctors and hospitals across the country that had been doing second trimester abortions cut back.

Once again, the victims are women.

*   *   *

And who are these women who seek late abortions?

Almost all of them are very young. They are minors who are afraid to tell their parents they are pregnant, until that pregnancy starts to show. Frequently they are children—thirteen, fourteen or fifteen—who refuse to accept the fact that they are pregnant until that fact is obvious to others. They are young people outside the information system, who live in communities where there is no one to turn to for information on early abortion.

If an older woman seeks a late abortion, and this is rare, she is apt to be someone in her forties, who thinks she is in menopause and discovers it is pregnancy. Or she may be someone who does not have regular monthly periods, and does not experience other early symptoms of pregnancy. Or she may be someone whose periods have continued after conception.

She may be a woman with mongolism in her family, or the woman who already has produced an abnormal child and wants to be sure the fetus she carries will result in a normal person. Tests for chromosomal abnormalities can be done, but not until about the fourth month of pregnancy. Then, after the test, a culture must be grown which may take another three to six weeks, and this woman may not know until her fifth month of pregnancy that she is carrying a retarded, deformed fetus.

Not long ago I was contacted for help for a sixteen-year-old girl who was near the end of her second trimester of pregnancy. Her father had a construction business, and a relative, a young man in his twenties, had come to work for her father and had stayed in their home until he found an apartment. He had raped the sixteen-year-old and she became pregnant as a result. She was afraid to tell anyone —she was afraid of the young man and afraid of her father. Finally, she told a teacher, who helped her tell her mother. These are the tragic stories behind the requests for late abortions.

In January, 1975, I spent many hours arranging a late abortion in New York City for a mentally retarded black girl from the Milwaukee ghetto. She was fourteen years old and had no idea of what had happened to her. Some man had taken advantage of her mental deficiency to impregnate her. Despite her tragic circumstances no help was available for her in Wisconsin, where the few hospitals that do a limited number of late abortions cut off at eighteen or twenty weeks.

No woman ever gets pregnant in order to have an abortion. No woman ever says to herself, "Well, I'm six weeks pregnant, but I'm going to wait and have my abortion at six months because it will be so much more fun." Women ask for late abortions for serious and compelling reasons, and the option of late abortion must be kept open for all these tragic cases.

# APPENDIX A

## *Types of Abortions*

THERE ARE THREE TECHNIQUES commonly used for doing abortions, and the kind of abortion a woman has depends on how far advanced her pregnancy is and how skilled her doctor is. Some physicians who accept patients for early suction abortion do not do later abortions. In general, the sooner an abortion is done the safer and simpler it is.

Most abortions in the United States are done now by vacuum aspiration. This relatively new technique is used up to ten weeks of pregnancy. A local anesthetic (para-cervical block) is injected around the cervix, which to some extent numbs the cervical and uterine area. If necessary, the cervix is enlarged by dilators (metal rods) although in very early abortion dilation is minimal. Next a small, flexible plastic tube about the size of a drinking straw is inserted through the cervix into the uterus—some doctors use a metal nonflexible tube. Then by means of gentle suction the contents of the uterus are removed through the tube into a collection bottle. The doctor then checks the uterine lining with a curette (a tiny instrument with a long handle and a spoonshaped end) to be sure that all tissue has been removed. This method, including giving the anesthetic, usually takes less than ten minutes. Most women experience some cramping during and after the procedure, similar to menstrual cramping, and this ranges from slight to severe. When the anesthetic is properly administered, most women can be kept fairly comfortable.

Women usually rest for an hour or so at a doctor's office or clinic before leaving, and are given things to eat and drink. It is advisable to rest the same day one has an abortion, but many women return to normal activity the next day.

There will be some bleeding for a few days following an abortion, and this may range from slight to heavy. Temperature should be taken daily as long as there is bleeding; many doctors routinely prescribe antibiotics to guard against infection. If someone has unusual cramping or clotting or heavy flow, she should stay in touch with her doctor, since this sometimes indicates that some tissue may have been retained in the uterus. In the event such tissue is not expelled, a follow-up D & C may be necessary.

It is a good idea not to have intercourse for two to three weeks after an abortion because of the risk of infection, and to shower, rather than bathe, as long as the bleeding continues.

The method of abortion used from ten to fourteen or fifteen weeks is dilation and curettage, in which the pregnancy and lining of the uterus are scraped away with a curette. This method requires more dilation than for vacuum aspiration, and has slightly more risk of perforation of the uterus. This technique can be used in a clinic or doctor's office up to three months, but it is generally done in a hospital after twelve or thirteen weeks.

Abortions beyond sixteen weeks of gestation are done by saline injection, or saltout. A long needle is inserted through a locally anesthetized area of the abdomen into the uterine cavity. Some of the amniotic fluid is withdrawn and replaced with an equal amount of a strong sterile salt solution. The salt solution causes contractions, and the fetus is expelled, usually within twenty-four hours. This method of abortion carries more risk than a D & C, and because it involves a two-day hospital stay, costs are high. Prostaglandins are being used instead of the saline injection in some hospitals.

Late abortions are done in some instances by hysterotomy, a miniature Caesarean section. Since this is major surgery requiring a general anesthetic, a relatively long convalescence, and leaves the woman with a sizeable abdominal scar, it is used only in those relatively rare situations where saline injections prove unsuccessful.

# APPENDIX B

## *Pat's Cartoons*

A PIONEER IN THE ABORTION REFORM movement who made dilatories out of the rest of us, Patricia Theresa Maginnis of California, entertains herself and her public with her social commentary cartoons. Reprinted here are four that deal with abortion. Collectors may like to know that they are available as postals—write Pat Maginnis, Box 21, San Rafael, Calif. 94901.

The first cartoon may need a little explanation for those unfamiliar with the abortion reform movement. To their great credit, a group of clergymen in New York City established the Clergy Consultation Service on Problem Pregnancies in the late 60's, counseling and referring women for abortions. The organization had clergy counselors in most of the major cities in the country by the early 70's, and their contribution to abortion rights in the United States was substantial. Two clergymen were arrested—one in Chicago and one in Cleveland—although the cases were later dropped. Others endured uneasy moments from police surveillance and phone taps.

Almost without exception the brochures and pamphlets of the early abortion reform movement, including those of the clergy, pictured a helpless woman with bent head and abject posture. Feminist Pat Maginnis turned those tables with a delightful cartoon.

93

WOMEN'S COUNSELLING FOR PROBLEM CLERGYMEN

Hominy Dominy Counselling Service
PO Box 6083 San Francisco, Ca, 94101

94

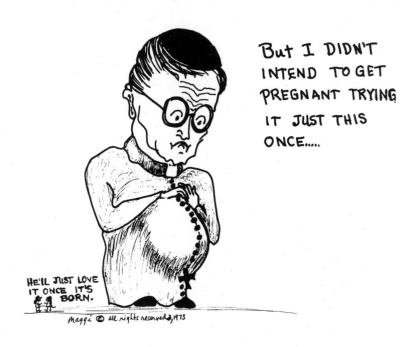

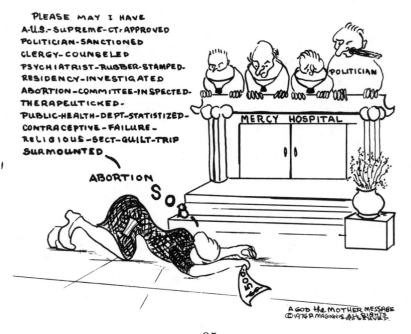

This next cartoon of Pat's could have been drawn to order. The week I received it I had talked at length to a waitress asking for abortion referral who had seven living children, ages twelve, eight, seven, six, four, eighteen months and three months. She had had three earlier pregnancies that ended in stillbirth or miscarriage. She was tormented by varicose veins, had had a blood clot, and her last labor had lasted two and one-half days. Her exhaustion was apparent, but she brightened a little during our conversation. For the first time in her life she was going to control a pregnancy, it wasn't going to control her.

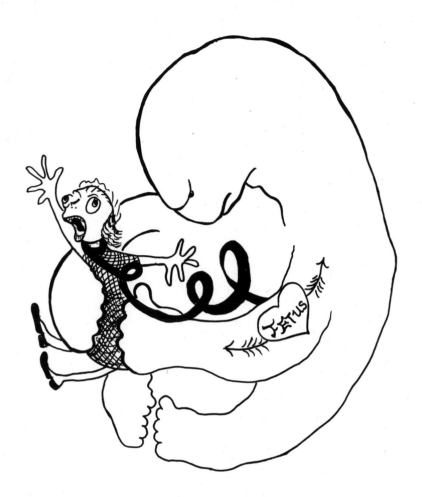

A GOD-the-Mother Message
© Pat Maginnis 1973, all rights reserved
P.O. Bx 21, San Rafael, Ca 94902

# APPENDIX C

# *A Bow to The Activists; Booby Prizes For The Obstructionists*

FOR THE PAST FEW YEARS the Wisconsin Confederation of Zero Population Growth has held annual awards programs to salute state pioneers in the birth control and abortion reform movements, and to bestow negative awards on particularly unhelpful types.

The first awards conference was held in Oshkosh in 1971 and Paul Ehrlich presented two awards: a Humanitarian Award to Dr. Alfred Kennan for "his courage and compassion in founding the Midwest Medical Center," and a Family of the Year award to the Richard Franz family of New Berlin for their activities in a variety of population and environmental causes and their two-child family.

Subsequent expanded programs were held in Madison.

Those honored in 1972:
| | |
|---|---|
| *Humanitarian Award* | Hania W. Ris, M.D. |
| *Activist Awards* | Edith Rein |
| | Lawrence Giese |
| | Gene Boyer |
| *Media Awards* | Appleton Post Crescent |
| | Nancy Heinberg, Capital Times |
| *Family of the Year* | James and Caroline Greenwald and daughters Elaine and Geraldine |

Those honored in 1973:
| | |
|---|---|
| *Humanitarian Award* | Rep. Lloyd Barbee |
| *Activist Awards* | Christine Correra |
| | Emily West |
| | Peteranne Joel |
| *Media Awards* | Whitney Gould, Capital Times |
| | Ron Carbon, WMFM |
| *Family of the Year* | Robert and Nancy Staigmiller and sons |

Those honored in 1974:
| | |
|---|---|
| *Humanitarian Award* | Herbert Sandmire, M.D. |
| *Activist Awards* | Rev. Elinor Yeo |
| | Beatrice Kabler |
| | Joan Allan |
| *Family of the Year* | Jeff and Jill Dean |

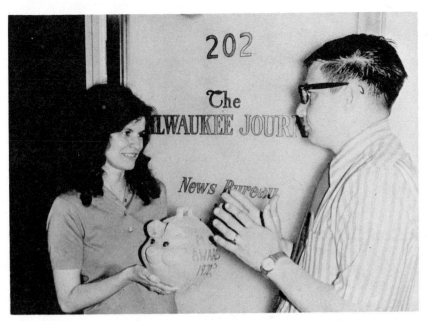

The *Milwaukee Journal* was chosen for a negative award in 1972 for its refusal to accept an ad for the ZPG Referral Service. It also was cited for its refusal to desexigrate its help-wanted ads, and for having a low number of women editorial employees. The *Journal* finally did drop the male-female distinctions in its help wanted ads, and reportedly has improved its percentage of female employees. However, in 1975 the *Journal* will not allow the words "abortion referral" in its advertising columns. It has editorialized that it is deplorable that some women still find their way to ghetto abortionists, but it will not consent to do the obviously helpful thing, and list non-commercial services that will give free information on where to go for safe, legal abortions. The only exception has been for the advertiser's willingness to use a euphemism such as "crisis pregnancy" or "problem pregnancy"; no reference may be made to abortion.

The *Journal* did not send a representative for its award, so I delivered it to their Madison bureau. Charley Friederich was on hand to accept the "Male Chauvinist Pig" Award.

101

A Wisconsin legislator from Darlington was selected for the booby prize in 1973. Gordon Roseleip, a flag-waver who likes women "in their place", was an adamant opponent not only of legal abortion but of any change in Wisconsin's anticontraceptive law. He uttered many memorable remarks during his years at the State Capitol including the award-winning pronouncement memorialized in the poster below. State Senator Roseleip was defeated for reelection in November, 1974, by a feminist, Kathryn Morrison, the first woman ever to serve in the Wisconsin State Senate.

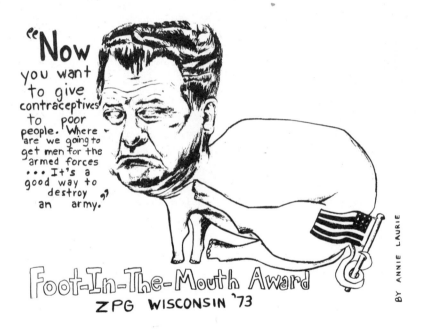

102

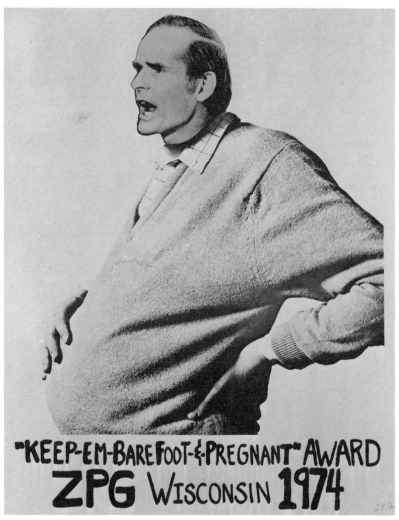

"KEEP-EM-BAREFOOT-&-PREGNANT" AWARD
ZPG WISCONSIN 1974

The senior U.S. Senator from Wisconsin, William Proxmire, announced his intention in December, 1973, of supporting an amendment to overthrow the U.S. Supreme Court decision on abortion, an action that brought him ZPG's negative award for 1974, a "Keep-em-Barefoot-and-Pregnant" poster.

# APPENDIX D

# What You Can Do

HERE ARE SOME SUGGESTIONS for activities.

Join the National Abortion Rights Action League (NARAL), 250 West 57th St., New York, N.Y. 10019. NARAL is the major national group working to protect and extend women's legal right to choose abortion. Besides its New York office, NARAL has a lobbying office in Washington D.C. and is one of the organizers of the International Association for the Right to Abortion, the first international abortion rights group formed at Bucharest in 1974.

NARAL members receive regular mailings which alert them to legislative happenings and court developments. Brochures, mounted photographs, and slides are available as aids to speakers. NARAL holds annual meetings in Washington D.C. and regional meetings around the country during the year. NARAL will put you in touch with groups and individual members in your state.

Support other organizations working to protect the Supreme Court abortion decision. Some of these are:

Zero Population Growth
1346 Connecticut Ave., N.W.
Washington D.C. 20036

National Organization for Women
1957 East 73rd St.
Chicago, Ill. 60649

Women's Political Caucus
1921 Pennsylvania Ave., N.W., Suite 300
Washington D.C. 20006

Association for the Study of Abortion
120 West 57th St.
New York, N.Y. 10019
(a tax-exempt source for information and reprints)

Women's Lobby
1345 "G" St., S.E.
Washington D.C. 20003

If you live in an area where abortion and sterilization are not available, make a fuss! Complain to doctors, hospitals, and your county and state medical societies. Check your state's maternal death figures for the past few years. In every state women have died because safe abortions were not available to them to end unwanted pregnancies, or sterilizations to avoid them. Publicize this information.

Arrange proabortion presentations in your area. Every little boondock in the country has been saturated with anti-abortion propaganda. Conduct your own educational campaign with the help of the following movies or others:

"Women Who've Lived Through Illegal Abortions"
c/o Planned Parenthood
810 Seventh Avenue
New York, N.Y. 10019

Aspiration Abortion
c/o Berkeley Bio-Engineering
1215 4th St.
Berkeley, Calif. 94710

In "Women Who've Lived Through Illegal Abortions" six women of different backgrounds and ages recount their experiences in coping with illegal abortions. Black and white, fifteen minutes long, this is an excellent movie around which to build a discussion. "Aspiration Abortion" is a twelve-minute medical film demonstrating the technique of suction abortion. A California gynecologist, Sadia Goldsmith, interviews a young woman patient and performs the abortion. The films are especially effective used together, since the horror stories of the "Women Who've Lived Through Illegal Abortions" contrast so sharply with the safe simplicity of the legal abortion, done for a composed patient in antiseptic surroundings with supportive people.

# APPENDIX E

# *Finding An Abortion*

ALTHOUGH ABORTIONS ARE LEGAL throughout the United States, their availability varies markedly from state to state. A woman seeking an abortion in Los Angeles or New York will have a variety of facilities to choose from, while the woman who lives in North Dakota or Louisiana may have no place within her state to go at all.

It is legal for any physician to perform an abortion, but problems arise in that very few American physicians have been trained to do abortions. Not only may a woman's gynecologist be unwilling to do an abortion, he may be inexperienced, and not a good person to turn to because he is unskilled. The suction method of abortion used during the first ten weeks of gestation is the safest, simplest method of abortion, but few specialists own the equipment or are experienced in using it. All gynecologists regularly do a dilatation and curettage (D & C) for diagnostic reasons, a method that is traditional for early abortion, but the procedure becomes trickier with a pregnant uterus, requiring more skill because of the increased risk of perforation.

Women who have no sources of referral within their own communities can phone the nearest Planned Parenthood clinic; most Planned Parenthood affiliates are reliable sources of information on where to go for abortions. Almost every college campus has a volunteer referral service, staffed by feminists, or at least a "hot-line". These can be found through listings in college newspapers or by phoning the student activities bureau. Chapters of the National Organization for Women (NOW) will have information, as do most Zero Population Growth (ZPG) chapters. Clergy Consultation Services on Problem Pregnancies have phone listings in some major cities.

If you have insurance, be sure to check it for possible coverage of abortion costs. Many policies have been expanded to cover abortion since its legality became totally clear. Women on welfare can use their medical cards for abortion care in many states. Costs for an early abortion vary, but if you pay more than $200 for a first trimester abortion, you are being taken. The going rate in New York City for an early clinic abortion is $125. On the west coast, charges average out in the $100 to $125 range. Chicago clinics charge about $150. A D & C done in a hospital will cost from $250 to $350, and a late saline abortion, with its average two days of hospitalization, costs anywhere from $350 in New York to $900 or $1,000 at some rip-off Midwest hospitals.

Confirmation of a pregnancy can be done by a simple urine test, if a woman is forty-two days from the first day of her last normal menstrual period. Most abortion referral sources will have information on where to go for inexpensive pregnancy tests.

# APPENDIX F

# The Tragedy of Tay-Sachs Disease

THE PROBLEM OF THE WOMAN who fears she may be carrying a fetus that has a genetic disorder has been touched on only fleetingly in this book. Kay Jacobs Katz, the mother of a child who had Tay-Sachs disease, testified before the Subcommittee on Constitutional Amendments of the Senate Committee on the Judiciary, on June 4, 1974. This committee, headed by Senator Birch Bayh, presently is considering the various antiabortion amendments proposed in Congress designed to write a ban on abortions into the U.S. Constitution. Excerpts from Ms. Katz's eloquent testimony follow.

My name is Kay Jacobs Katz of Silver Spring, Maryland, and I am the mother of a child who had Tay-Sachs disease. I appear here today to express my personal beliefs and to represent the National Capital Tay-Sachs Foundation, an organization committed to public education, cure research, health care and prevention of Tay-Sachs disease and its allied disorders. These genetic diseases, known as sphingolipidoses or lipid storage diseases, are characterized by inborn errors of lipid metabolism. In each disease, an enzyme necessary for normal human function—hexosaminidase-A—is either deficient or inactive, resulting in neurological deterioration and early death. It is estimated that one in every thirty American Jews of Eastern European ancestry is a carrier of this trait. A carrier is totally unaffected by the disease, but a blood test can determine that the amount of activity of "hex-A" is somewhat less than that of most individuals. Statistically, one in every 900 Jewish marriages is between two carriers, who are therefore capable of producing a child with Tay-Sachs disease. One child in every 3600 births to Jewish couples will be afflicted with Tay-Sachs disease, and every child born with this disease will die by the age of four. . . .

There are a great many people who wish to deny potential parents of infants with fatal genetic disorders the option to terminate affected pregnancies. However, once a doomed baby is born, these same people who insist on his birth disappear, leaving total responsibility to his parents. Besides the heartbreak, mental anguish, and, quite frankly, physical burden that the parents must endure, there is the problem of finding people willing or qualified to help in caring for such a child.

In most cases the families seek out institutionalization at some point, because of increasing medical problems or simply overwhelming demands on the parents' time. Most retardation centers are inappropriate, and hospital-care costs are prohibitive. Most insurance companies refuse to cover prolonged hospital care on the basis that it is custodial care—even though the medical profession disagrees. Even those insurance companies that do cover a prolonged hospital stay will not cover the cost of a nurse at home, which for many families would be a much more acceptable form of help. . . .

It all started for us four and a half years ago when we had our first baby. She was beautiful and, we were assured, healthy and normal. She grew and developed very normally for several months—or so we were told. There were a few little problems, such as a pronounced startle response which she never outgrew, but the doctor reassured us that she was normal. By ten months of age she had begun to grow weak and to lose some of the skills she had learned, and once again I pleaded with the pediatrician to tell me what was wrong. Again, as before, I was put off. Finally, a couple of weeks prior to her first birthday, he admitted that her development was not progressing normally, and we were referred to a specialist at Children's Hospital here in Washington. We brought Joann home the day before her first birthday, with the knowledge that she had Tay-Sachs disease, that the birthday cake placed in front of her the next day would be the only one she would ever see, and that she would no doubt be dead before her fourth birthday.

We made every effort possible, for Joann's sake, to continue to provide a normal environment for her. As she continued to lose skills and awareness, we adapted our life style and care of her to her needs. I took her for physical therapy and learned the exercise program myself, so I could prevent stiffness from taking over her body, as she moved about in her crib less and less.

Although we made a valiant attempt to believe that a cure would come along in time to save her life and restore some of her intelligence, each passing week took more and more away from her. So as not to dwell on her deterioration, I will summarize by stating that by the time she died on May 28, 1973, she was a blind invalid, seizuring and drowning in her own secretions, requiring daily enemas, naso-gastric feeding (fed a liquid diet via a tube plunged down the nose into the stomach), and spending more time in oxygen and on antibiotics than not. These were the very real events we had to stand by and helplessly witness, and when you love someone the way we loved Joann, you would do anything to reverse the insidious process that was taking her away from you, and short of that, anything to prevent its recurrence.

When Joann was diagnosed, we learned that Tay-Sachs disease is an incurable degenerative disease of the nervous system, uniformly fatal by the fifth year of life; beyond all that it is hereditary. Not only was it going to kill my daughter, it would mean that if I were to conceive again, there

113

would be a 25 percent chance of any fetus being affected with the disorder.

We learned that in the case of this particular genetic disease, and a growing number of others, prenatal diagnosis was now possible, and that if the fetus in question were affected, safe, legal termination of the pregnancy was also possible. We had a big decision to make because we desperately wanted more children of our own. After several months of soulsearching, we decided to go ahead and plan a second pregnancy. I refused to become pregnant, in other words, until I was convinced that there was no hope for Joann, and that I would have the courage to undergo an abortion rather than produce another Tay-Sachs baby. Besides her own short, hopeless life, there remained the fact that we had established a love relationship with Joann before her illness became apparent. With a subsequent baby we would know from the day of his birth of the possibility of his impending death, and could never have given him the same loving kind of care we gave Joann, and feel we owe our children. At some point the instinct of self-preservation forces one to protect oneself from pain.

Therefore, when I did become pregnant, I was referred to a physician specializing in genetic counseling who saw Joann and discussed her with me, and who later met with my husband and me to explore our attitudes and feelings, and to make sure we had all the pertinent information we needed. He assured us that he himself would be performing the prenatal test known as amniocentesis; the necessary cell cultures would be grown in his laboratory and sent for analysis to the National Institute of Health. If the results were unfortunate, he would perform the abortion himself and stay with me afterwards, to be supportive and help in any way possible; for he knew how hard it would be for us, but also understood why and how we had made such a decision.

All this information is really background material to help you understand why we feel so strongly that by depriving couples like us of the option of having children unaffected by such serious and hopeless disorders, you are

114

really depriving us of having children at all. Most of us would simply not be foolhardy enough to knowingly risk a pregnancy without this alternative. We now have a healthy, normal two-year-old son, and we expect another baby free of Tay-Sachs in July. If an anti-abortion amendment is passed and ratified, I will be one of the lucky few who had the freedom to have such a family in the few short years while the medical and scientific capability was available and legal. . . .

Tay-Sachs is only one of a number of related disorders; it is also the most common. For parents of children suffering with some of the related diseases, there is as yet no prenatal diagnosis, and these couples are anxious for medical research to find the means to make it available, so they too may have children with a fair chance for survival. However, because of the cutbacks in funding for medical research in this area on one hand, and the threat of an antiabortion amendment on the other, these couples would have to give up hope of having more children. . . .

I know that the subject of Tay-Sachs disease has come up previously before this subcommittee, and that the suggestion has been made that two known carriers simply not marry each other. This idea rings of the same simplistic reasoning that I have heard again and again in antiabortion thinking. This is not the beginning of time; marriages between carriers already exist. My husband and I are an example of this. Would it suit society's needs better if we dissolve our marriage, to avoid having children together? Not only is the argument simplistic, it is fallacious. A couple who decides against marriage because they share one of 2,000 currently identifiable lethal genes might separately marry someone else with whom they share the potential for some other genetic disease in their offspring, as it is a well-established medical fact that each of us carries between five and ten such traits. Simplistic, fallacious, and even unreasonable is this idea, because the law would then be denying individuals a very basic human right in our society—the right to marry the person of one's choice. And so once again we confront the conflict of exactly whose rights are to be protected, those of the fetus or those of the couple who conceived it.

Were safe, legal abortions unavailable, we would be caught in a vacuum offering few alternatives. We do not believe that abortion is a "cure-all," or a matter to be taken lightly. We realize only too well the seriousness of the situation and we dislike the reality that termination of pregnancy, and late in the second trimester at that, is the only means we have of achieving normal families. We would much prefer a cure, and for this reason my husband and I, with the support of family and friends, have established a small research foundation in our daughter's name, to keep cure research alive. However until successful therapy is possible, we will continue to fight for the right of couples to terminate pregnancies that would otherwise bring them heartbreak.

It would seem also that banning legal abortion would force us to undergo sterilization operations, because no means of contraception is totally effective for everyone, and we wish to avoid having doomed children. If we are faithfully practicing birth control, and our method fails us, we are then forced to bring a child into the world whose life and death will break our hearts, or forced as in earlier days to become criminals in the eyes of the law and seek abortion where we can find it.

I have great respect for the United States Senate, but I do not believe that its members are more qualified than I to decide on the question of abortion. I believe that it is such a personal, complicated, and difficult decision for everyone who approaches it, that no legislation concerning it could really satisfy all its aspects. Difficult though the decision may be, I have the right to make that decision for myself and I want that right preserved. I refuse to sit idly by and watch pressure groups exert their influence on my government to erode my rights as an American citizen, and I implore you and your colleagues to reject these efforts in favor of the individual freedom upon which our society is based. . . .

# APPENDIX G

## *Extracts From The Supreme Court Decision on Abortion January 22, 1973*

From the Texas decision (Roe v. Wade):

1. A state criminal abortion statute of the current Texas type, that excepts from criminality only a *life saving* procedure on behalf of the mother, without regard to pregnancy stage and without recognition of the other interests involved, is violative of the Due Process Clause of the Fourteenth Amendment.

(a) For the stage prior to approximately the end of the first trimester, the abortion decision and its effectuation must be left to the medical judgment of the pregnant woman's attending physician.

(b) For the stage subsequent to approximately the end of the first trimester, the State, in promoting its interest in the health of the mother, may, if it chooses, regulate the abortion procedure in ways that are reasonably related to maternal health.

(c) For the stage subsequent to viability, the State, in promoting its interest in the potentiality of human life, may, if it chooses, regulate, and even proscribe, abortion except where it is necessary, in appropriate medical judgment, for the preservation of the life or health of the mother.

2. The State may define the term "physician," as it has been employed in the preceding numbered paragraphs of this Part XI of this opinion, to mean only a physician currently licensed by the State, and may proscribe any abortion by a person who is not a physician as so defined. . . .

This holding, we feel, is consistent with the relative weights of the respective interests involved, with the lessons and example of medical and legal history, with the lenity of the common law, and with the demands of the profound problems of the present day. The decision leaves the State free to place increasing restrictions on abortion as the period of pregnancy lengthens, so long as those restrictions are tailored to the recognized state interests. The decision vindicates the right of the physician to administer medical treatment according to his professional judgment up to the points where important state interests provide compelling justifications for intervention. Up to those points the abortion decision in all its aspects is inherently, and primarily, a medical decision, and basic responsibility for it must rest with the physician. If an individual practitioner abuses the privilege of exercising proper medical judgment, the usual remedies, judicial and intraprofessional, are available.

From the Georgia decision (Doe v. Bolton):

4. The three procedural conditions . . . violate the Fourteenth Amendment.

(a) The JCAH accreditation requirement is invalid, since the State has not shown that only hospitals (let alone those with JCAH accreditation) meet its interest in fully protecting the

118

patient; and a hospital requirement failing to exclude the first trimester of pregnancy would be invalid on that ground alone. . . .

(b) The interposition of a hospital committee on abortion, a procedure not applicable as a matter of state criminal law to other surgical situations, is unduly restrictive of the patient's rights, which are already safeguarded by her personal physician. . . .

(c) Required acquiescence by two copractitioners also has no rational connection with a patient's needs and unduly infringes on her physician's right to practice. . . .

5. The Georgia residence requirement violates the Privileges and Immunities Clause by denying protection to persons who enter Georgia for medical services there. . . .

# APPENDIX H

# *Abortion Around the World*

THE ABORTION REVOLUTION is spreading around the world and many countries recently have modified age-old restrictive laws. Here is a partial summary of the status of abortion in various countries as of early 1975.

## GREAT BRITAIN

Many American women flew to London for abortions prior to the legalization of abortion in New York. It has been a haven also for women from the religion-dominated countries on the European continent.

Great Britain first legalized abortion through a 1967 Act of Parliament, which permits abortion if continuation of the pregnancy involves a risk greater to the woman's physical or mental health than termination of the pregnancy. Two doctors are required to approve the procedure which can be done for the first twenty-eight weeks of pregnancy.

## SWEDEN

The first liberalization of Sweden's law occurred in 1938, but the law remained restrictive, gradually being

121

amended and broadened, but still involving immense amounts of red tape. In January, 1975, most of the bureaucratic hurdles were abolished, and women now may have abortion on request through the twelfth week of pregnancy. There are special formalities still required for second trimester abortions.

## FRANCE

Although stormy discussions about abortion are continuing in France, the French National Assembly, after a prolonged televised debate, voted on Nov. 29, 1974, to legalize abortion on request at set prices during the first ten weeks of pregnancy. The new law went into effect on Jan. 18, 1975. It is regarded as a stunning triumph for feminists in this heavily Roman Catholic country.

## ITALY

In February, 1975, Italy's constitutional court decreed that a woman's right to health and sanity took precedence over an embryo, which the court described as "not yet a person." Several proposals for abortion reform have been submitted to the Italian Parliament, with the issue still being debated in early 1975. Estimates of the numbers of illegal abortions in Italy have varied from the Ministry of Health's 800,000 to the three million estimate of a 1968 convention of Italian gynecologists. The World Health Organization estimates 1.5 million annually.*

## WEST GERMANY

The West German parliament passed a law permitting abortion during the first twelve weeks of pregnancy in June, 1974. The law did not go into effect, awaiting a Supreme Court ruling which was handed down in February, 1975. The Court ruled that the law violated a constitu-

*New York Times, (March 23, 1975) pp 1, 53.

tional principle that "everyone shall have the right to life and inviolability of person."

The verdict angered many Germans. Almost 60 per cent of them, in national polls, had expressed themselves desirous of a change in the restrictive law, and the negative court decision triggered large demonstrations in most German cities.

## SPAIN AND PORTUGAL

Abortion remains illegal in both of these impoverished nations. Attacks on abortion are common in the press and on television, which is state-owned. Feminists are a rare breed, and the reaction in these countries to the liberalization of the abortion law in France was one of shock.

## SWITZERLAND

For decades Switzerland has had the reputation of being the place to go in Europe for well-to-do women who could afford illegal abortions at luxurious clinics catering to the rich.

Swiss women themselves never were so lucky, and a country that only very recently gave women the vote still is debating her right to an abortion. In March, 1975, the lower house of the Swiss Parliament narrowly defeated a government bill that would have legalized abortions for other than grave medical reasons.

## EASTERN EUROPEAN COUNTRIES

In most of these socialist countries abortion has been legal and free since shortly after World War II. Laws have become more restrictive in a particular country when male leadership is in the throes of a population expansion drive. The concept of abortion as a woman's right, resting with her and not with the state, is not grasped too well around the world, even in those countries that have experienced decades of abortion legality.

## SOVIET UNION

Abortion was legalized in Russia in 1920, but under Stalin it was prohibited again, except for grave medical necessity. In 1955 a woman's right to abortion was reestablished through her first trimester of pregnancy. Russian women may get time off from employment for abortions, and be paid for the abortion if they obtain a medical certificate to present to their employers. In Moscow alone there are an estimated 200,000 abortions per year, about twice the number of births.

## SOUTH AND CENTRAL AMERICA

Abortion remains totally illegal in almost all of South and Central America, although illegal abortions are commonplace. These are performed by midwives or witch doctors in shantytown huts or country shacks. The wealthy may be accommodated in clinics or private hospitals. In San Salvador, the capital of El Salvador in Central America, one admittance in every five at the maternity hospital is for a woman who is having complications from back-street abortion, a typical situation throughout Latin America.

Abortion is permitted legally in Argentina in those cases where a woman's health is jeopardized seriously, or a fetus is known to be retarded or deformed. Since the Peronist government in Argentina is desirous of doubling the country's population by the end of the century, there seems little likelihood of further liberalization of its law. In fact, a decree has been issued restricting the sale of oral contraceptives and, in general, discouraging all methods of birth control.

Probably the weirdest liberalized abortion law in the world is that of Uraguay. The law, notable for its double-talk and its view of woman as a chattel, reads in part:

(1) if the offence [meaning an abortion] was performed to safeguard the honour of the woman or that

of her spouse or a close relative, the penalty is reduced by one-third to one-half; the judge may totally exempt the parties concerned from punishment in the case of abortion performed with consent, after an examination of the circumstances of the case; (2) if the abortion is performed without the consent of the woman in order to terminate a pregnancy resulting from rape, the penalty is reduced by one-third to one-half, no penalty being imposed if the operation is carried out with the woman's consent. . . .*

Serious danger to health and serious economic difficulty also are recognized by Uraguay's abortion law, with or without the woman's consent!

## JAPAN

Abortion has been legal for twenty-seven years in Japan, and a woman may obtain one through the seventh month of pregnancy.

Since Japan had no tradition of contraceptive use, and its feudal family system meant inequality for women, the permission for abortion was not granted with women's rights in mind, but strictly as an economic measure. At the end of World War II destitute Japan was a nation of seventy-two million persons. In the four years following the war it added eleven million more. Struggling for economic survival, the Japanese knew they must do something to control a population fast outgrowing area and resources, and they first liberalized abortion in the late 40's and, after a couple of years' experience, extended the law to accommodate abortion on request. Within ten years from the first liberalized law, their birthrate was cut in half.

Contraception has become more available in Japan since the advent of abortion. In the 1920's birth control crusader Margaret Sanger had been denied entry to Japan, and twenty-five years later General Douglas MacArthur again refused her request to enter. Tokyo's largest paper

*World Health Organization, *Abortion Laws: A Survey of Current World Legislation,* Geneva, WHO, (1971), p. 26.

reported, "In view of the pressure of the Catholic Church groups, it was believed impossible for General MacArthur to allow her to lecture to Japanese audiences without appearing to subscribe to her views."* At that time in Japan there was a Catholic population of 130,000, in a country of over eighty million people.

## THE EAST

Abortion and birth control both are available to Chinese women, as a health service without charge. In India, a law passed in 1971 gave Indian women the right to obtain hospital abortions. Unhappily, hospital facilities are available only in the cities and 80 per cent of Indian women live in villages. In the Middle East abortion remains strictly illegal, even in Lebanon, the most sophisticated of these countries, where no abortions are performed even to save a woman's life.

## AFRICA

Early in 1975 the all-white South African parliament passed a bill providing that a woman may have an abortion only after obtaining certificates of necessity from three doctors. In a special racist touch, the bill stipulated that a pregnancy may be ended if it is the result of sexual intercourse between a white and nonwhite, an act forbidden by law in South Africa. In most of Africa abortion is seldom mentioned and remains illegal, although in major cities it is available for those who can afford the fees.

## CANADA

Abortions have been allowed in Canada since 1969 when necessary to preserve the life and health of a woman. A committee of three or more physicians must agree to the

*Emily Taft Douglas, *Margaret Sanger: Pioneer of the Future*, (New York: Holt, Rinehart & Winston, 1970), p. 247

necessity, and the procedure must be done in a properly accredited hospital.

In 1973 Dr. Henry Morgentaler, who worked in a poor neighborhood of Montreal, was arrested after having performed some 2,000 abortions in a clinic setting, pioneering the suction method in Canada. He was acquitted by a jury, but this decision was overthrown by the Quebec Supreme Court. Early in 1975 the Canadian Supreme Court by a 6-3 decision upheld the Quebec court. Dr. Morgentaler was sent to prison to serve an eighteen month sentence in Montreal.

Although Canadian law allows abortions for life and health reasons, only some 250 of Canada's 1,000 hospitals have abortion review committees. Much of Canada is without any facility a woman can apply to for abortion care, even to save her life.

Therapeutic abortions approved by committee are covered by Canada's National Health Insurance, and such abortions continue to be quite readily available through the hospital committee route in cities such as Toronto and Vancouver. Again, women with contacts and money to travel may get abortions: others may not.

Dr. Morgentaler's case is believed to be the only case in Canadian legal history where a jury acquittal was overthrown by the Canadian Supreme Court. Canadians working for women's freedom to choose abortion now have no recourse through their courts. Their goal is to convince their national Parliament to remove abortion from the criminal code.

DATE DUE

MAR 1 7 2006

NOV 2 9 2006

ILL: 32674276
DUE: 4 WEEKS USE
NO RENEWALS

MAR 17 2014

DEMCO, INC. 38-2931